Doctor, Stay By Me

Reactions to Doctor, Stay By Me

"This marvelous, real and heartfelt series of gripping and poignant stories is a joy to read. Dr. Stafford Cohen's fifty-year journey through his honest and expert service to patients is an important personal history of how medicine was in its most kind and 'patient' era, a humane description that implicitly warns against the billing machines of our day that seem to turn our sacred calling into profane work. All health-care workers—and patients—should read it to chuckle, be touched, and inspired."

Samuel Shem, M.D.
Author of The House of God *and* The Spirit of the Place.
Professor of Medical Humanities at NYU Medical School.

"Stafford Cohen is a very gifted writer. He provides enough description (but not too much) to place the reader right next to the patient and the patient's immediate surroundings. The book is a gem and it will be greatly enjoyed by everyone fortunate enough to read it."

N. Paul Rosman, M.D.
Professor of Pediatrics and Neurology,
Boston University School of Medicine.
Division of Pediatric Neurology,
Boston Medical Center.

"After reading Dr. Cohen's book—I must say, 'Bravo.' It is beautifully written, with such heart, wit and, most importantly, great empathy. I love that it gives a fascinating almost voyeuristic glimpse into the world of medicine. The last story about Duke has haunted me, so terribly sad, but the reality of medicine today."

Martha Hall Kelly
Author of the acclaimed novel, **Lilac Girls.**

"For me it is a page turner. I especially enjoyed reading about the Munchausen patient—as I have dealt with that kind of very challenging situation. In general it is wonderful—as Dr. Cohen takes the reader across all segments of humanity as he makes his point about the privilege that we have of knowing people so intimately as we try to help them."

Gail Metcalf, Nurse Practitioner
Extended Care Community Practice (ECCP).

"I found the stories to be absolutely engrossing—the prose was both eloquent and clear. More specifically, as a younger physician reading through the book, I found the stories to be hopeful and aspirational. I, like many of my peers, went into medicine due to a love of patients and patient-care. The stories affirmed this unique privilege of being a physician and allowed me to reflect on both the wonderful patient relationships that I have developed through medical school, residency, and fellowship and the times when I missed opportunities to develop stronger relationships. I also thought over and over about the impediments to relationship building and how I can ensure that I overcome these impediments in my future practice."

Robert M. Stern, M.D.
Hematology-Oncology Fellow,
Dana-Farber Cancer Institute.

"I really enjoyed these cases and found many of them quite moving. They raise interesting and important issues that all physicians need to think about."

David S. Jones, M.D., Ph.D.
A. Bernard Ackerman Professor of the Culture of Medicine,
Faculty of Arts and Sciences and the Faculty of Medicine,
Harvard University.

"This captivating collection of clinical vignettes will appeal to both the medical and non-medical reader. Thoughtful analysis by a humanistic, compassionate cardiologist. The 'art' of medicine dominated his career. Listening, observation, compassion and empathy were essentials of his physician-patient relationships.

"Now an M.D.'s attention is diverted by the explosion of data, technology, shortened clinic visit time, the computer in the exam room, excessive regulatory requirements and emphasis on the financial bottom line. Has the pendulum swung too far from the 'art' to the 'science' of medicine—from time to tech? Do we need a new balance?"

Gretchen Rooker, M.D.
Internal Medicine (Retired)

By Stafford I. Cohen, M.D.

Paul Zoll, MD
Doctor, Stay By Me

Doctor, Stay By Me

A medical memoir about the era before the forced fracture of the patient-doctor relationship, and its needed repair.

Stafford I. Cohen, M.D.

Copyright © 2019 by Stafford I. Cohen, M.D.
All Rights Reserved

Without limiting the rights under copyright reserved above, no part of this publication may be reproduced, stored in or introduced into a retrieval system, or transmitted, in any form or by any means (electronic, mechanical, photocopying, recording or otherwise), without the prior written permission of the copyright owner.

For reasons of privacy, the stories have been altered and the patients, precise times and places have also been disguised. In many instances, the patient is a composite of several patients.

Opinions regarding the practice of medicine and its delivery of care contained in this book are those of the author and not those of the administration of any of the medical institutions that the author
has ever been affiliated with.

Cover photograph of the author by Bachrach
is used with permission.

"A Dying Man's Wish Fulfilled"
This article first appeared in the Texas Heart Institute Journal: August 2016, Vol. 43, No. 4, p. 285-286.
© 2016 Texas Heart® Institute, Houston.

"Jim's Prostate Cancer"
This article first appeared in the Texas Heart Institute Journal: February 2017, Vol. 44, No. 1, p. 9.
© 2017 Texas Heart® Institute, Houston.

First Edition: 2019
Printed in the United States of America.
ISBN: 9781793176974

To Deborah

The Front Cover: A Handshake

A traditional handshake is the most common greeting in the western world. It is far more prevalent among men than women. The custom might have originated 900 years B.C. when an Assyrian King is depicted shaking hands with a Babylonian leader. In Ancient Greece and Rome, a handshake was symbolic of friendship, and in Medieval Europe it was evidence that an unclenched fist did not have a weapon. For centuries, a handshake "sealed the deal" between parties of an oral agreement, and in modern times this ritual became an important non-verbal act that communicates good will.

The cover of this book depicts a traditional introductory greeting between a doctor and a patient. Their handshake is a simple symbolic act that defines their relationship. The doctor will do no harm and agrees to be an uncompromising advocate. The patient agrees to be truthful and trusting of the doctor.

Just as the time honored patient-doctor bond has weakened and its importance devalued in the current model of clinical care, so too the traditional handshake is being replaced by "high fives" and "fist bumps"—especially among the younger generations. Alternative greetings are in vogue throughout our country and appear to be a form that was instituted just for thoughtless fun.[1]

End Note

1. The "high five" and "fist bump" greeting might have a hygienic advantage. Hands harbor and spread microbes. That granted, the traditional handshake should be maintained in the doctor's office and the hospital to help reinforce the mutual importance of the patient-doctor relationship. Hand hygiene is not an impediment to a handshake, for doctors are instructed to hand wash before and after each patient encounter and each patient should have access to a wash basin and a bottle of hand sanitizer while at the doctor's office or in the hospital.

Table of Contents

Acknowledgements 1
Prologue 3
Introduction 7

Chapter One — Medical School
Introduction 9
Act of Charity 11
House Call #1 12
House Call #2 16
Marine Biology and Research 19
A Medical Student in London 25

Chapter Two — Know Thy Patient
Introduction 33
The Immigrant 34
Once I Was Strong 37
The Man of Mystery 40

Chapter Three — Spirituality and Belief
Introduction 51
Denial 52
May God Guide Me 57
Caught Between Two Sciences 59

Chapter Four — Always Ask a Patient about their Pet
Introduction 62
A Grateful Patient and a Show Dog 63
Service Dog 65
A Dying Man's Wish Fulfilled 67

Chapter Five — Near the End of Life: What Gives Meaning to Life?
Introduction 70
A Patient's Dilemma 73
The Master Watchman 77
The Greek Sea Captain 81
Jesse 84

Chapter Six — The Tyranny of Guidelines
Introduction 88
Jim's Prostate Cancer...92
A Patient without an Advocate 94
Doctor, Treat Not Thyself..97

Chapter Seven — Directives
Introduction 101
Assault and Battery..102
When Good News is Bad News 109
Going Express..113

Chapter Eight — The Pathologist Doesn't Always Have the Last Word
Introduction 115
Cancer, Where Art Thou?..117
Circumstantial Evidence..119
See No Evil, Speak No Evil, Hear No Evil 123

Chapter Nine — Suicide
Introduction 127
Attempted Suicide—Ad Seriatim 130
Change of Heart 134
To Err is Human...138

Chapter Ten — Futility
Introduction 142
An Unexpected Request 143
Will to Live..146
We Believe in Miracles..148

Chapter Eleven — Holocaust
Introduction 150
To Life 151
When the Heart Stops Beating...155
Underground 158

Chapter Twelve — Weddings
Introduction 169
Tradition 171
A Matter of Honor 174
Damaged Goods 177

Chapter Thirteen — The Good Death
Introduction 180
Contemplating an Honorable Death 181
A Socially Acceptable Death 184
A Good Doctor and His Good Death 188

Chapter Fourteen — Regrets
Introduction 191
Unintended Consequences 192
Sacrificed for the Greater Good 196
Duke 199

Epilogue 205

ACKNOWLEDGEMENTS

I extend my gratitude to those who contributed time, effort and ideas that helped me craft this book.

They follow:

Bernard Mendillo, who guided the first draft to the final publication of this book.

The reviewers, in alphabetical order:
David S. Jones, M.D.
Martha Hall Kelly
Gail Metcalf, NP
Gretchen Rooker, M.D.
N. Paul Rosman, M.D.
Samuel Shem, M.D.
Robert Stern, M.D.

PROLOGUE

"Change is inevitable."

Fortunately, that aphorism applies to advances in medical science, diagnosis and treatment. There has also been change in the delivery of medical care. The initial change was gradual, then the rate accelerated and then there was a gathering storm of scientific technical breakthroughs, out-of-control costs and the application of business principles to enable medical care to be profitable while maintaining a satisfactory margin of patient safety.

I have no experience as a social engineer or as an innovator in public-health policy. But in my 51-year immersion with delivering care to patients, and as an observer of trends in medical education and doctoring since my retirement from patient care 11 years ago, the patient-doctor relationship has been devalued. In retrospect, I realize that I was fortunate to have cared for patients when there was time to develop strong relationships with them. Patient-and-doctor time together is the crucial ingredient that enables a satisfactory relationship; but current time constraints have weakened that bond. Abbreviated visits, the interposition of nurse practitioners and technicians, medical teams[1,2] and medical-related technology have isolated or separated the patient and their primary doctor from each other. Judicious and short-term separation might be beneficial, but overuse is harmful. Gadgets permit patients to self-monitor vital signs, sleep patterns, exercise metrics, heart rhythm, oxygen saturation and other parameters. In addition, there are many Internet websites where a person can gather medical information or remotely interact with a previously unknown nurse or doctor in a manner that qualifies the person as a patient based on a check-box questionnaire and/or a conversation. The unexamined newly coined patient can then receive a prescription for a powerful medication. Detractions that erode the doctor-patient relationship will be a constant theme throughout this book.

In the current atmosphere, neither my past patients nor I could enjoy a satisfactory relationship. There has been a degradation of that valued interaction—that tight bonding—with my patients that I had previously been able to uphold. Today it is estimated that half of doctors and a large percentage of patients are unhappy with their caring and their care. Both doctors and patients can look for change. Doctors can transfer their skills to other institutions that will permit more time with patients—a giant step forward to repair their frayed humanistic goals. Likewise, unhappy patients can seek out a member of the endangered species of primary-care doctors that are empathetic and more interested in their patient's welfare than their employer's interest, the medical insurer's interest or their own self-interest.

I was fortunate to have practiced in a medical center that allowed me to organize my own time. That was in the past and would not be possible today. Since retiring from patient care, I miss the patients. I often reflect on numerous memorable patients and their problems. I decided to write about their stories and our relationship. The thread of their true story and our relationship was imbedded in memory, so there was no need to gather their records for documentation. For reasons of privacy, the stories have been altered, and the patients, the times and the places have also been disguised. In many instances, the patient is a composite of several patients. During my 51 years of direct exposure to literally thousands of patients in about 16 separate institutions,[3] disguising a patient's characteristics and circumstances (except the main thread in the fabric) was easy.

The honesty of the patient-doctor relationship is what distinguishes a medical career from all others. In its current vitiated state, it should be repaired and maintained.

It is my hope that readers of this book will have a greater appreciation of the limitations that the current system imposes on their doctors and the allied health specialists that are entrusted with their care.[4]

Stafford I. Cohen, MD
Newton, Massachusetts
2019

End Notes

1. Bellafiore G. 23 hours and 23 people: a patient's perspective. Heart Rhythm 2017; 14(1): 149-150
2. Boycott KM, Innes AM. When One Diagnosis Is Not Enough. N Engl J Med 2017; 376:83-85
3. Opinions regarding the practice of medicine and its delivery of care contained in this book are my own and not those of the administrations of any of the medical institutions that I have ever been affiliated with.
4. I have no financial disclosures such as financial conflicts of interest or commitments relating to this book

INTRODUCTION

In the best of times, whenever and wherever doctors encountered patients, the doctor was a shepherd to a sick member of their flock through the natural course of an illness. By custom, they treated their patients at home, in the office or in the hospital. They stayed by their patient, whether the infirmity ended in recovery, debilitation or death.

Doctors were committed to their community, found satisfaction in their mission, were united in a professional code of ethics and generally behaved within the spirit of the ancient Hippocratic Oath.

In modern times, the patient-doctor relationship has deteriorated for a number of reasons. Because of powerful forces it is unlikely to greatly improve.

Where do we stand today?

In my opinion, it is not possible to provide high-quality care if patients are placed on the moving belt of an assembly line that has its rate increased by invoking the necessity of adhering to ever changing business practices. To be sure, some business directives for shorter visitation times are essential if a medical entity is to survive financially. But to quote a well respected principled colleague who elected to retire from practice in favor of industry because he would not compromise on quality: "If there is a financial loss on each service, higher volume will not solve the problem."

The stories that follow occurred when there was time for patients and doctors to bond. Although the pace of medicine was advancing at the time of these stories, the pace was slow enough for doctors to care about their patients and for patients to have confidence that their doctors would stay by them.

CHAPTER ONE
Medical School

Introduction

During the first year of medical school, I soon became comfortable with the academic routine except for the Gross Anatomy Course, which was a torturous rite of passage during the transition from learning about the body's superficial exterior to understanding its mysterious sacrosanct interior structures that underpin the vitality of life. The cadavers were unclaimed or donated "teachers." Their autopsy-dissection had the dual purpose of determining a cause of death and educating student prosectors. Kidney cancer had dealt our "teacher" its fatal blow. The right kidney was a mass of solid tumor which obscured its normal anatomy. My partner and I had to peek at the opposite kidney after a pair of our classmates had exposed its essential parts. The experience of surgical dissection was transforming for our entire cohort as we took a giant step towards obtaining our goal of being accepted into the ranks of a time-honored special profession. I did not possess exceptional surgical skills, so the anatomy lab experience dissuaded me from being a surgeon. That opinion was reinforced, as I struggled to stay awake at 4:00 A.M. while holding retractors during an emergency operation.

Compared to classroom lectures and book learning, the out-of-classroom activities were new, challenging, mind expanding—and a growth spurt in understanding the multiple roles open to a medical doctor. The clinical rotations were new and unfamiliar. They demanded being in a "doctor-patient relationship," and being a participant in a story that had a beginning, analytic component and a resolution; in other words, a patient's chief complaint, examination, formulation of a diagnosis and a treatment plan.

As a novice, I saw many unexpected acts of charity, made house calls during a community-medicine rotation, participated in a basic research project during a summer vacation and had an externship within a socialized form of health care in England. Those transforming experiences that follow occurred in medical school and remain vivid in memory.

Act of Charity

Most of my medical and surgical-clinical rotations were at a major teaching hospital for the underserved, where cafeteria-style, free, buffet meals were provided to hospital personnel. Qualified workers entered a moving line while selecting and placing items on their tray. At the exit, a rotund, jovial, red-headed inspector checked everyone's identification and stamped their meal card. I usually arrived just minutes before each closing. Occasionally, grimy, unkempt persons in tattered clothes preceded me in the lunch line and exited without showing an identification or meal card. The apparent interlopers were never the same, but their general appearance was undeniably similar. One day, I managed to get through the line behind one of these unusual people. So I asked the enforcer, "How come I notice that you didn't check the person in front of me or other similar appearing folks. Do they work here?" He told me to come back after I finished my lunch, because that's when we would have time to talk privately.

As instructed, I met with him a while later.

"You have an untrained eye for spotting the homeless folks in this impoverished neighborhood," he began. "Some are alcoholics, some are mentally ill, and others are down on their luck. Most are hungry, undernourished and in a state of semi-starvation. Haven't you noticed? They're all thin."

He paused, looked about to be certain that no one was listening, and took a deep breath before continuing. "Without a balanced meal, they end up semi-conscious on the street, are gathered up by the police and admitted to this hospital where they stay for a while before discharge. Then the cycle starts over again. I try to break the cycle by giving them a square meal. Either way, the city pays and it's a lot less for a meal than a hospitalization. That's the answer to your question. Now think about it and be on your way."

I thought about it, and realized that I had been taught a lesson in life that made sense. That day I learned more in the cafeteria about acts of charity than on the medical ward—where the lunch-room-warden's actions would have fallen under the rubric of preventive medicine.

House Call #1

The Community Medicine course required making house calls within the impoverished, high-crime community that surrounded the medical school. After the last home visit of the day, each case was presented to the instructor and my cohort back at the classroom. So we proudly assumed the role of real doctors as we dressed in a short white coat and carried a black doctor bag. In those days, doctors were given a free pass by the neighborhood thugs to assist residents in trouble. We had the uniform and played the part. In later times, anyone in such a uniform would invite being victimized by gang members who expected that the signature black bag contained drugs.[1]

My first assignment was to see a 20-year-old woman with abdominal pain. She was new to the system. Her uncle called in the complaint, phone number and address—32 Main Street, second floor. When I arrived at the address, a sixth sense alerted me that something was wrong. This was a commercial area. Number 32 was bracketed by a bar and a pool room. Perhaps there was living space on the upper stories. After the door to 32 opened with a twist of the knob, I stepped into the entryway. A pay phone with the intake number was on a wall to my right. It was surrounded with paper messages held by thumbtacks. There were also three, keyed mailboxes —all belonging to business firms. A long flight of stairs was dead ahead.

The place was silent, so I called out, "Anyone home, anyone here?"

A shadow appeared at the landing above.

"Doc, is that you? Come right up. You're at the right place."

During the ascent, a singular thought kept reverberating in my mind: "This isn't going to be a classic house call."

After arriving on the upper landing, I was greeted by a dark-complexioned man named Joe. His gray-felt hat and oversized overalls seemed out of place. I was led through a grated open door into a dimly lit empty loft with a freight elevator at the far end. The only furnishings were a few wooden chairs. One was occupied by a thin short man, named Uncle Jim, dressed in a well-pressed dark suit, a straw hat, white leather shoes and sunglasses. Behind him was a red curtain suspended on a wire between two poles that were about eight feet tall.

Neither man said a word. So I ventured, "Where is the patient—the woman with the painful abdomen?"

Joe pulled back the curtain exposing a girl covered with a sheet, lying face down on a sagging cot. She turned her head and stared at me with huge, wide-open, white-saucer-like eyes, each with a brown-rimmed dilated central pupil. Were they an expression of fright? Of concern? I introduced myself and asked about her name. When she did not reply, Uncle Jim did —"Samantha." I then asked Samantha to describe her chief complaint and her present illness. Again, there was no reply.

I tried another approach. I told the gentleman that I would be examining Samantha and for the sake of preserving proper amenities and privacy, to draw the curtain and move a good distance away. That accomplished, she answered my questions in a hushed voice. The problem started with a vaginal discharge that continued for four or five days. Then there were shaking chills, drenching sweats, nausea and abdominal pain.

Pertinent findings on examination revealed fever, rapid heart rate, a tense upper and a tender lower abdomen.

To my question about being sexually active, Samantha answered with one whispered word, "Yes."

My sixth sense was correct; this was neither a house call nor a house in the true sense of the word. I stated my diagnosis, prognosis and treatment to this strange trio. Samantha likely had gonorrhea-induced pelvic inflammatory disease, and was in need of a gynecological examination and intravenous antibiotics in a hospital.

Uncle Jim strongly objected to a hospitalization. He wanted me to prescribe antibiotic pills. Under the circumstances, I did not have the authority to do so and knew that my supervising doctor would not do so. I reiterated the need for hospitalization. I told Uncle Jim that he had two choices, either transport Samantha to a hospital by automobile or transport her by ambulance. He agreed to transport her in his automobile. Uncle Jim said, "Thanks;" Joe was mute; and Samantha's hand barely waved. I left, returned to the classroom, gave my report and was told by the instructor that no student had ever made such a convoluted house call. He requested that I try to learn what finally happened. What was the follow up? So I rang up the telephone at 32 Main Street. There was no answer on three consecutive days.

Finally someone answered. "This is Sam, what's the good word?"

I asked for Joe, Uncle Jim or Samantha.

"Who? Never heard of them."

Then the phone went dead.

End Note

1. Today, doctors and health-care workers who make house calls in unsafe communities blend in with the crowd. They wear street clothes and carry their medical tools in a backpack.

Stafford I. Cohen, M.D.

House Call #2

At a later time, during the course in community medicine, I was assigned to see Mrs. Adalia Holt, a 65-year-old diabetic with a complaint of a stubborn cough. The intake information indicated that she was a widow who lived on the second floor of a three-family, brownstone walkup. To gain access, I was told to ring the bell of the first-floor neighbor who had a key to Mrs. Holt's apartment. That arrangement was required because she spent most of her time in bed or in a chair. It was hard for her to get around. A long-term diabetic, Mrs. Holt had suffered the ravages of that disease. It had caused legal blindness (while retaining partial vision), cardiovascular and peripheral vascular disease with more than one heart attack, and a below-the-knee amputation of the right leg.

There was a chill in the air when I set out from school for the patient's home visit. Upon arrival, my exhaled breath formed a frosted vapor while walking up the half-dozen steps to the entry. Everything went as planned. I was escorted to my new patient's front door. The apartment was sparsely furnished. Every wall had peeling paper. The place was warmed by two, small, steaming, upright iron radiators on either side of the bed's high headboard. Mrs. Holt was propped up with her back pressed against it. The room was dimly lit by a single naked ceiling bulb and a few rays of sun that shone through a solitary window that had a long crack in the upper glass panel. On one side of the bed were a wheelchair, commode and a table. The bed had an overhead trapeze arrangement and an abbreviated bed rail to assist Mrs. Holt when changing her position. On the other side of the bed were a long, round, thick stick and a crutch. Both were within arm's length. I settled into an empty chair on the opposite side and faced Adalia Holt. Her large arthritic hands were folded across her chest from which a short neck supported her head topped with long gray hair. Her face featured large brown eyes and a mouth adorned with bright-red lipstick. Her hands abruptly moved from chest to mouth to stifle a paroxysm of coughing. She then pulled a tissue from a box on the bedside table and blew her nose. The surface of the table held several other items including a small mirror, a radio, a telephone and a hammer.

The history and examination were most compatible with a viral upper-respiratory infection. Symptomatic treatment was recommended, such as Tylenol for fever, cough suppressants, hydration and close management of diabetes.

I was curious about Mrs. Holt's current circumstances and "way of life." She had no children. Her husband had worked for the city sanitation department before dying in his 40s from a stroke. Financial security (or perhaps insecurity) was in the form of welfare, subsidized housing and food stamps.

I asked, "How do you spend your time?"

"Mostly listening to the radio."

"Do you talk to friends on the phone?"

"No, the phone costs too much. It's only for emergency 911 calls."

"Well then, what do you do if you need some non-emergency help?"

"We have a system here. I alert the downstairs neighbor who let you in by pounding on the floor with this heavy stick."

To be sure that I knew what she meant, her index finger pointed to it.

Then she picked up the hammer from the table and shook it while saying, "If I need the upstairs neighbor, I pound on the radiator. The pipes go straight up there. Do you see where the corner radiator paint is chipped? I did that."

She smiled and looked so pleased until she coughed a few times before going on.

"I'm not lonely or dependent," she continued. "My arms are strong. I can transfer to my commode or wheelchair and take care of myself. If my arms or shoulders hurt, I can rest them against one of the hot-water steam pipes. I can heat my food in the kitchen. A nurse checks on me each Tuesday and an aide bathes me each Thursday. Lord knows, friends and neighbors drop by all the time. I hope that you're able to come again. Stop by next week and see how I'm doing. I'll tell you more about our community and how we support each other."

I learned more about resiliency, life and communal caring from Mrs. Adalia Holt than about her common upper-respiratory viral infection. Unfortunately, my rotation changed within the week so I could not return for a followup visit. But I later learned from a classmate that she had fully recovered.

Marine Biology and Research

I received a message from Dr. Paul Larson, the professor of physiology, to meet at his office after class. My first inner thought was, "Had I failed the most recent examination?" Luckily there wasn't an academic problem; the dark side of my imagination had worked overtime. Larson, in a blue shirt with rolled-up sleeves, was pacing about his office. When he sat down, his parts continued to move. Chewing gum kept his face and jaw changing in a vertical direction and the upper leg that crossed over the lower was in constant diagonal motion.

He explained his agitation. His two-part research grant was finally approved to study why sea urchins shed their eggs and the mechanism by which starfish discard an injured appendage. The first is important for survival of the species, the other for individual survival. Grant approval came late, after its initial rejection was appealed on grounds that the project had commercial value. A robust market for tastily prepared sea-urchin eggs had emerged in Japan with the potential to destroy the sea-urchin resource. Perhaps eggs could be harvested while preserving the life of its host—if so, the resource would be renewable and sustainable. The starfish project was a harder sell regarding its commercial value. Starfish are predators of clams and other shellfish. Owners of some Maine and Canadian private islands leased areas of shoreline for aquaculture. The beds, seeded with clams and mussels, were harvested by a formula that would sustain the resource. Any information about starfish behavior should be welcomed, especially methods of keeping starfish far from shellfish farms.

With final grant approval in Larson's hand, an immense amount of preparation was required. The experiments would be performed at a marine biology lab in Maine. Larson said it was a terrific place in general and a better place to work. He had spent many past summers there. But the schedule was "tight" with only eight weeks to prepare. Larson then stopped chewing, looked me straight in the eye and said that I would have right of first refusal to work in the laboratory as a research assistant. Room, board and a small stipend would be provided.

That's how I was introduced to scientific research.

After completing personal preparations and a lot of administrative paper work, I settled in at the research lab. My job description wasn't rigidly defined. Drew Pitcock was my co-research-fellow. He was an upperclassman who had worked with Larson in the past. We cleaned and stocked the lab, washed the glassware and made sure that the continuous saltwater spigots and drains, essential for our specimens, were in working order.

Dr. Larson was a brilliant teacher. His lectures demystified complex subjects and made them crystal clear for the dullest of dull students. During the summer, I learned that Larson was sparse on scientific publications at the medical school, and on the last grant application his important sources of research funding at the school were not approved. Paul Larson was on probation. His university appointment was in jeopardy. The adage, "publish or perish," was a reality. He was still treading water, in imminent danger of sinking, and he was not happy. Meanwhile I was having the time of my life.

The research was fun; the community was intellectually stimulating with lectures on the most fascinating subjects—like the chemistry of phosphorescence, which is how sea creatures light up in the dark, or how salmon find their way back to their birth place in freshwater streams after spending years in the open ocean.

In addition to this exciting work, we had Nobel Prize recipients like James Watson give lectures. He helped identify the DNA double helix. Also, there were many opportunities to relax. Take your pick—beaching, boating (that had been Larson's choice), fishing, tennis, bridge and enough musically inclined personnel to field an orchestra. Let me not forget the many fun-loving investigators who frequently organized late-night parties.

Larson had a small bungalow on a five-year renewable lease that was owned by the marine-biology lab. The lease was contingent on his academic appointment there, and his remaining in good standing. The lease could be unilaterally terminated for any reason at any time. He and his second wife, Sandy, intermittently had us over for a cookout. Larson's first wife was Lorraine; she had died six years earlier from cancer; and they had no children. The bungalow was on a low-grade upward incline in front, perched above a steeper downward incline in the back. There were flower and vegetable gardens on each side of the pathway that descended from the rear door to a lower-level patio with its charcoal grill, picnic table and benches. Heavy rains had eroded and deeply crevassed the soil. Sandy and Paul Larson were optimists. They believed that a terraced slope would remedy the erosion and enhance the property for their enjoyment when, and if, he was able to extend the lease. Towards that goal, large wooden railroad ties were stacked at the side of the driveway. Drew and I were conscripted to drag them onto recently prepared trenches for the terracing. Not in our job description, but hard to refuse our host before or after a great cookout that was a welcome break from our institutional-style fare. An added attraction was a spectacular seascape view of the harbor, some islands beyond and an open expanse of ocean that was impinged upon by a swerve in the distant mainland.

Larson was always high strung as each cookout got underway. He was the chef; the coals had to be just right before committing an entree to the grill. At his home, Larson was a chain smoker which was probably the reason he chewed gum elsewhere. After a drink of Scotch, he would calm down and, after a couple more drinks, would tell us great stories about his adventures while tracking the habits of sea creatures like giant squid and octopi from the polar regions to the equator. They were the subject of his master and doctorate theses and they continued to be his special area of scholarly marine expertise; whereas, at the medical school, he researched renal physiology with comprehensive knowledge about the human kidney's countercurrent exchange.

On a memorable evening after the cookout and placement of railroad ties, we relaxed to watch the sun set without Sandy. She had retired to the bungalow. As Larson spun another high adventure sea story, the western sky was transformed to a glorious red sunset that reflected on a Maine-made Friendship sloop under full sail. Larson, with Scotch in hand, stopped speaking in mid-sentence. He drained the glass, changed the subject, and launched into a tirade. He chastised the majority of doctors for losing sight of their mission to preserve their patients' health. Doctors should assiduously serve their patients. Practitioners and specialists, whose opinions are valued, earn their reputation by committing all their energy to learning the science of illness and the art of care. After achieving local or widespread fame, some believe they are important. They parlay their reputation into entrepreneurial enterprises that detract from patient responsibilities. Larson paused, pointed a gnarled index finger at us saying, "Don't let that happen to you! Forget about fame and fortune!" He picked up the bottle of Scotch, refilled his empty glass, and then resumed his monologue.

"Do you see that sailboat down there? I had one just like that. For many years, Lorraine and I often sailed from here during the day while I ran the lab experiments during the evening and night. We spent favorable-weather weekends sailing along the coast. Sailing was our pleasure. But it resulted in our accumulating a hell of a lot of direct and indirect reflective sun exposure. Lorraine noticed a dark "mole" on her upper arm and saw an eminent dermatologist. It was biopsied. After receiving no word from his office, we assumed that all was well. Five months later, Lorraine noted swelling and pain in her arm pit, not too far from the biopsy site. We returned to the famous dermatologist."

Larson paused, put his glass down, lit a cigarette and took a deep drag.

"The swelling was from enlarged lymph nodes. One was biopsied. It revealed malignant melanoma with the same cell structure as the original biopsy five months earlier. Our superstar dermatologist had spread himself so thin that he neglected to carefully review the damming original biopsy report on his desk. He had patented a proprietary formula for a psoriasis cream that launched a business. As the president, he was often on a speaker's circuit. As a matter of fact, he left on a lecture tour the day after Lorraine's original biopsy. When he returned, he just filed her report away. That error was Lorraine's death sentence."

Larson's eyes became moist. He wiped away the tears with the back of his free hand and regained his composure.

"After she died, I sailed our boat single-handed. It was designed that way. While alone in the boat, I constantly reflected on my many, many, happy memories with Lorraine. The fact that they should have been ongoing made me angry. That's an understatement—it made me furious—and intensified my depression. I was, and still am, unforgiving. So I reluctantly sold the boat to lessen my grieving."

Day was yielding to night. We cleared the picnic table, said our farewells and departed. Drew and I reflected on Larson's sad tale and vowed to be responsible to our medical mission and to our patients by upholding our modified Hippocratic Oath to the letter. We were condemned to "Do No Harm."

Our research was fruitful. We learned that sea urchins can shed their eggs when stimulated by a weak electrical current. Starfish shed an appendage when exposed to an as-yet-unknown protein that originates from damaged neural tissue. We started to "moth ball" the lab in preparation for the fast-approaching academic year. I received a message that Paul Larson wanted to meet with me the next day over lunch. Once again my first thought was, "What did I do wrong this time?"

We met in the cafeteria. Larson's message was mixed. The collaborative renal-research grant submitted by the medical school had not passed muster at the National Institute for Health. Larson, a member of the cobbled-together research team, was now without any funds. His status with the medical school went from probation hell to unadulterated hell. In a lowered voice, he explained, "My lectures will be given by a bright young investigator with a large grant to identify new substances using chemical column chromatography. I've heard his terrible presentations. Any student will have to be a genius to understand him. The school is sacrificing your education for this clown's grant money. He should be confined to the lab and be barred from the classroom. If you have trouble with his lectures, contact me and I will give you a copy of mine. At your stage, you should be made aware of the insecurities of academia."

After Larson stopped to clear his throat with a couple of swallows of lemonade, I thought to myself, "What a shame."

Larson proceeded with the other half of his mixed message by asking me to join him next summer at the marine lab. I was not sure about plans for my last remaining summer vacation before starting an internship. The medical school had encouraged my class to expand our horizons by spending an externship abroad. Dr. Paul Larson accepted my gratitude for being honored by his offer and he understood my inability to commit. We finished lunch. Before leaving, he popped two sticks of spearmint chewing gum in his mouth.

Working at the marine biology laboratory exceeded my expectations. Executing a research plan was exciting and fun. It was a transforming experience that would be a strong influence for me to consider a career in academics.

A Medical Student in London

I was late, en route to morning rounds at St. Bartholomew's Hospital. On the final lap, through the Smithfield district wholesale meat markets, workmen were clearing the street of straw, of melting blocks of ice and of discarded extraneous animal parts. Long narrow carts with large wheels carried sides of beef, slaughtered sheep, and unidentified carcasses hanging on huge hooks attached to overhead bars. The carts clogged the walkway while awaiting transfer of their cargo to one of the many wholesale meat markets that lined both sides of the street. A few delivery vehicles were being loaded with produce on one side. High, great glass overhanging arches on either side partially enclosed the street, but left a vertical vent along its length. The arches further dimmed an already dull-gray day, but thankfully permitted the loading and unloading of produce during drenching rains that were so common to London. I abruptly hopped into the gutter in mid-stride to avoid a pushcart that appeared from nowhere, tripped over a severed pig head and toppled to the ground. Never saw the pig head, as I intently eyed the advancing pushcart heading straight toward me. The pusher never stopped; he just kept going. I righted myself, dusted off, and proceeded lickety-split toward the hospital, after assuring myself that only my pride had been hurt. On days to come, I successfully avoided other wayward pig heads as I rushed through Smithfield.

I was lucky to be accepted as an extern at a London hospital during my last-ever, summer class break. St. Bartholomew's Hospital (St. Bart's) was an austere place. It was founded in 1123, on the site of a religious revelation. Many members of its medical and surgical staff had made their indelible mark in the annals of medical history. I was familiar with three before I got there. I knew of surgeon John Hunter's classic description of his angina pectoris, Percivall Pott's discovery that scrotal cancer in chimney sweeps was an occupational hazard, and William Harvey's classical description of the cardiovascular system.

In 1960, London was still recovering from the massive bombing blitz inflicted on its patriot populous during WWII. Structurally unsafe, condemned buildings were awaiting demolition more than a decade after the war. The domed roof of Saint Paul's Cathedral was still undergoing repair. I sensed the war-time terror of the patients and staff every time I approached St. Bart's heavily pock-marked, bomb-gouged, stone-walled perimeter and entrance facade.

Within, my assigned patients were selected from two, open, all-male medical wards. Each had thirty fully occupied beds and a "private" room to insulate the ward population from disruptive psychotic screamers or from the disruption of the near dead on the way out. There was a hospital-based culture dedicated to boosting patient moral and comfort that far surpassed anything that I had seen in the US. The wards had spacious, beautiful wooden floors with perimeter heating grates and high ivory-colored walls. The two outer walls had windows that stretched toward the ceiling through which entered sunlight to brighten the ward and uplift the spirits of the ill. A nursing station, in the middle of the ward, was the responsive control center to the unpredictable ebb and flow of human suffering. The gentle nurses, officially designated as "Sisters," ran the wards. From their central vantage point, nothing escaped their swivel-headed sharp eyes. When they cranked open the windows, curious sparrows entered with the fresh air, became the focus of the ward as they flew about, and always proved to be a therapeutic diversion for those bed-bound patients who were traumatized or depressed by their circumstances.

The rear of the hospital grounds had spacious gardens, pathways, trees and manicured grass lawns that were maintained by volunteers. Personnel transported patients on their beds from the inner hospital to this tranquil space and back. At the side of each pathway were roofed, open-faced shelters to protect bed-bound patients from sudden rain showers.

Each ward had patients with a general mix of diseases. Diabetes, cancer cardiovascular and liver disease were the usual suspects. Our group of seven students was from the United Kingdom of Great Britain and its former colonies. I was the sole exception. My cohort's approach to learning was casual and undisciplined compared to my classmates in the US. Each in our group was assigned a patient to interview, examine, analyze the laboratory data, review the literature, formulate a diagnosis and present the case if called upon. The patients were cooperative and were treated by all medical and paramedical personnel with dignity and respect. Care was provided free-of-charge by the National Health Service. Doctors, Sisters and hospital workers were underpaid civil servants with a common mission—to care, comfort and cure the ill.

The practice of medicine was low-tech. There was a high regard and reliance on an impeccable history and physical examination, rather than a practice by some doctors in the US of performing a superficial inspection of the patient and ordering multiple tests. For example, at St. Bart's, when there was a question of thyroid disease, a dozen symptoms and signs were each given a weighted score of one to five. The extremes of the cumulative score pointed to overactive or underactive thyroid function. At home in the US, several different blood tests would be performed to establish or confirm thyroid malfunction, none of which were available at St. Bart's.

After one of our student group presented a case to the instructor and admitted that he was unsure of the abdominal physical findings, the instructor had the student get on his knees by the bedside, joined him on the spotless clean floor and demonstrated how a superior abdominal examination should be performed—not by looking and feeling from above, but by sitting or kneeling at the same level as a supine patient. I never witnessed the knees-on-floor approach in the US.

All the students in my group were cordial. One, William Worth, who preferred to be called Bill, was more than cordial—he was friendly. Bill appeared to be a little older and wiser than the others; older and wiser because he was repeating several courses after failing his examination for promotion to the next class. He was skinny, had crooked teeth, and had wire-rimmed eyeglasses. On many occasions, Bill spontaneously invited me for afternoon tea at his nearby lodging when activity on the ward had slowed to a near standstill. Bill wanted to learn about life in the US. His family was well off and he had the financial ability to travel abroad. He spoke of applying for further training in the US after securing his medical degree. Bill's father was an obstetrician. But Bill would not follow in his father's footsteps, because he didn't believe the specialty was very challenging. Bill said, "Why specialize in something that nature does well without any help? If nature needs help, a midwife can fill in. Perhaps trauma or wound healing or rehabilitation would be more appealing. Nature needs help with those problems."

Bill's parents lived in London near Russell Square. He was the youngest of five children. During the war, his oldest brother was killed in France, his other brother was crippled by a land mine and his two sisters drove ambulances for their hospital's emergency flying squads until war's end. Bill believed that he needed a lodging central to the university and hospital that would permit efficient use of time and a total commitment to study. His lodging was spacious and was in stark contrast to mine. Limited finances restricted me to a walk-up tiny living space that included a mini-kitchen, bathroom with a wash basin, and a room that served for living, dining and sleeping. There was a common bathtub half a flight down. Hot water for the bath, kitchen sink and bathroom wash basin was controlled by a coin meter, as was heat for the living space. Bill resided in a middle-income area. I lived in low-income Holloway, best known for its women's prison. Bill could walk to class or hospital whereas I hopped a bus, transferred at the train station and walked through a commercial area, before it merged with Bill's territory. I stocked my larder with peanut butter, jam, margarine, bread, milk and eggs. Bill had access to upscale restaurants and sidewalk cafes, whereas my neighborhood had an automat and some pubs. I developed a taste for pub food and drink. My favorites were fish, chips, and warm beer; or warm beer, pickled eggs and pigs' knuckles.

Bill's plans got sidetracked after he became romantically involved with a classmate. When she left him for an upperclassman, Bill totally lost his ability to concentrate and his mind went blank for hours whenever he caught sight of her.

The British medical educational system is less regimented than ours. Bill told me that whenever students believe they're ready for advancement, they notify the medial school. A date is set for written and oral examinations. Bill did well on the written set, but failed the oral exam.

He angrily remembered the examiner's first question: "Who first described the swollen lymph nodes behind the ears that accompany African sleeping sickness?"

"I forgot," Bill said, "that it was Thomas Masterman Winterbottom. That's all the bloody bugger examiner had to hear, so he bombarded me with questions about tropical diseases. My weakest subject—of course I failed."

During afternoon tea, we learned a lot about our different cultures and a lot about our shared ideals. I came to believe that we were members of a worldwide brotherhood with a common mission to "heal on demand."

The Sisters, who ran the wards, were highly experienced. They taught students how to perform procedures like blood draws from difficult veins, lumbar punctures (sampling spinal fluid), thoracentesis (sampling chest fluid), and paracentesis (sampling abdominal fluid). They encouraged the slow learners by telling them that with patience, time and practice, there would be improvement, and they rewarded the fast learners with a tea biscuit.

I noted that Sisters and doctors displayed equal compassion for all their charges, but there were two exceptions.

The first was a thirty-ish German woman on vacation who was admitted in the middle of the night with a seizure disorder. The hospital beds were totally occupied except for one in a private room on our all-male ward. During the war, the seizure lady had sustained a head and brain injury when struck by a collapsing section of a bombed-out building in Berlin. Seizures resulted from that injury. The war's residual effects left every member of our hospital staff with unhealed emotional wounds. Wounds like the bomb-related gouges that remained on the outer walls of the hospital. When the staff and my group of students gathered outside the German woman's private room, the lead doctor quietly said, "It's ironic to care for someone whose government tried to kill us and destroy our country. When they failed, they send us their citizens for free health care." The staff appeared to have no sympathy for the visitor. She was on the low end of the compassion scale. The staff increased the anti-seizure medication, added a low dose of another and advised immediate return to Germany for further care.

*

Rodney Hall was at the high end of the St. Bart's compassion scale. I learned a little about him by overhearing some chatter on the open ward. He was a 40-year-old, blond, blue-eyed, fair-complexioned, freckle-faced, former Royal Air Force (RAF) fighter pilot. The poor devil had Hodgkin's disease. He was here on an experimental chemotherapy protocol because he hadn't responded to conventional therapy. After the war, he taught aeronautical engineering and the history of air transportation at an elite private military-preparatory school. He was single. His older and younger brothers died during the war in the service of their country and their Majesties, the King and Queen. During the war, his mother and father died in a car crash when they were hit head on by a sleep-deprived British soldier on leave who was speeding back to his station. At St. Bart's, Rodney Hall was without visitors. He had no family, and his many friends and surviving air-force buddies were at a distance. There were no telephones available to the patients. Hall did receive bundles of mail from friends, but that was a poor substitute for an in-person visit.

St. Bart's permitted daily visitation hours from 4:00 P.M. to 6:00 P.M. during the break between the completion of all patient ministrations and the dinner meal. I was amazed at how disciplined the visitors cued up at their designated hospital entrance, each with a bouquet of home-grown flowers in hand. Each visitor was on a mission to cheer up someone in need. At 6:00 P.M., these missionaries quietly evaporated from the wards. Yet I noticed that any one of a number of Sisters always came to chat with Rodney Hall at his bedside at the start of visiting hours and always placed fresh flowers in a blue vase on his end table. The other item on the table was a framed photo of a man in uniform standing beside a fighter plane.

I also overheard one of the night-duty, senior medical trainees mention that just before lights out, a nurse-sister always stopped by Hall's bedside to learn if he was comfortable and had any complaints or needs.

I was not assigned to Hall's case, nor were any of my cohorts. What was his story? Why was he a Very Important Person (VIP) worthy of very special treatment? So I asked Sister Christine, a middle-aged, kindly, soft-spoken angel with a plump waist line. (She once gave me a tea biscuit after supervising my cleaning and suturing the lacerated arm of a motorcyclist who had crashed.)

She told me that Hall was an RAF Spitfire fighter pilot who had distinguished himself during the Battle of Britain. He was an Ace, a title earned after downing at least five enemy planes.

Sister Christine looked toward the ceiling as if she were witnessing his plane in flight, and then continued her story.

"His luck ran out. Any German Messerschmitt fighter plane was superior to a British Spitfire. Our boys were at a disadvantage. Rodney was in a prolonged dog fight over the Channel; enemy fire came through the cockpit, shattered his left leg and partially disabled his plane. His squadron buddies drove off the enemy Messerschmitt while our hero headed for the safety of home. Luckily he got close enough before bailing out, just before his plane spiraled in flames into the frigid Channel. Close enough that he was plucked out of the water by the captain of a small fishing boat that set out on a rescue mission after seeing the descent of the parachute. The captain got to Hall before he became critically compromised from extreme hypothermia and blood loss from nasty bullet wounds in his left leg. The frigid Channel brine likely saved him from bleeding to death by constricting the punctured vessels."

Sister Christine paused and asked herself, "Where was I?"

She answered her own question.

"Oh, now I know. You asked why we treat him so well. Remember, Americans were spared the brutality of war. Your country was not invaded. You were not bombed day after day. You did not freeze for lack of fuel. You did not burn every stick of furniture in your fireplace to stay warm. Your innocent citizens did not starve or freeze to death. I could go on, but let me get back to Rodney Hall.

"He spent a year in a military hospital because he had infected bone in his shattered leg and needed at least four reconstructions. He also had to emotionally cope with losing all members of his immediate family. Fighter pilots are tough, optimistic and resilient. Somehow, God knows, they bounce back. He had a gimpy leg, needed a lot of rehab; took to a crutch, then a cane. Hall got along with a bad limp that caused him to bob 30 degrees with each left step. Resilient—you bet. He wanted to re-enlist. He was turned down and appealed on the basis that he didn't need his left leg to pilot a Spitfire. The Force turned him down again, explaining that he had done more than enough for his country.

"Rodney Hall is my hero and my countrymen's hero. The men in the Air Force saved me, my family and my country. Our RAF pilots held off the enemy during the Battle of Britain. I know that, and Winston Churchill knew that when he said that Britain would have been defeated if not for their bravery and sacrifice."

Christine ended with, "So, my friend, that's why we believe he is so special. We encourage him to remain hopeful, because we are hopeful that he will be cured. But we and he know that the final outcome is in God's hands."

CHAPTER TWO
Know Thy Patient

Introduction

Most patients seen by an internist or cardiologist are old and ill. Too often, they are dependent because of physical or mental impairment. Doctors either treat the illness within the context of the person, or the person within the context of the illness. With either approach, we ask, "Who is the person that I am treating?" We physicians, and others in direct contact with our patients, realize that they have had a long journey and are a product of nature, nurture and innumerable experiences fused together by life and living. Each patient's "who" is a composite that will continue to evolve as long as they live.

Our task is to learn about each person who has honored us by seeking our advice. At times, that knowledge is difficult to extract, but the reward is worth the effort.

The Immigrant

The 72-year-old Asian gentleman, new to my practice, had an air of distinction as the receptionist escorted him into the consultation room. His approximate height was five feet, five inches. His body straight, head held high with a crown of neatly trimmed below-ear-length gray hair. A made-to-order, cuff-linked shirt with the initials T.N. embossed on the left breast pocket. A perfectly fitted, unbuttoned, light-blue suit and highly polished black-leather shoes embellished his image. Tommy Nu slowly glanced about the office then turned his head to greet me with half-smiling un-parted lips.

The referring doctor demanded that I see Mr. Nu as soon as possible because his patient complained of exertional shortness of breath. The primary-care doctor was too busy to answer any but my most basic questions about Mr. Nu's symptoms. The doctor told me that recent encounters and past records would be faxed that day. Mr. Nu would call for an appointment.

Although I gestured for Mr. Nu to be seated, he waited until I settled myself into my swivel chair. During the comprehensive history, he answered each question directly, with understandable precision, and with total command of the English language. Unbeknown to me, at the time, he was fluent in five languages.

I decided to delay the social history because that segment of patient information, documented at a prominent medical center in California, had near total redactions other than Nu's undergraduate education in Europe and his graduate studies in public policy at the John F. Kennedy School of Government in nearby Cambridge, Massachusetts. None of the subsequent medical records addressed his social history.

Pertinent review of systems revealed coronary risk factors of high blood pressure, peripheral vascular disease and previous heavy tobacco use which during the recent decade had become moderate. There had also been past significant pulmonary problems with several bouts of pneumonia. The tobacco habit and pneumonia led to a current diagnosis of emphysema.

Physical examination substantiated high blood pressure, peripheral vascular disease and emphysema.

I concluded that the symptom source was from either pulmonary or coronary pathology. After Mr. Nu walked about the office with an oximeter clipped to his finger that had recorded constant normal oxygen levels, my favored diagnosis became coronary artery pathology with an atypical presentation.

I suggested lifestyle modifications, prescribed new medications, ordered an imaging exercise study and scheduled a followup appointment to discuss the results of the forthcoming exercise study and to learn if there had been a change in symptoms.

Before Mr. Nu departed, I delicately asked him about his redacted social history. Once again he smiled without parting his lips, and then he said, "I requested that part of the record be eliminated, but I will speak about it if asked. Very few doctors have inquired."

I interrupted the storyteller while reflexively attempting to crush a fly that settled on my desk top. Having failed in the execution, I apologized and asked Mr. Nu to continue.

"I am the oldest child of a privileged family. After my formal education, it took 20 years to work my way up the political ladder of my country before I secured the top job as Head of State. My country flourished. Life was good, perhaps too good. Some in my trusted circle became envious and I was deposed in a military coup. My life was in danger as well as the lives of some members of my family. We left with our most valued possessions—our lives."

After a brief pause, his facial features remolded into a stern expression, he rose from the chair and paced to and fro, three or four steps at a time before he stopped, looked down at me and said, "Do not record what I am about to tell you."

I nodded in agreement. Then Mr. Nu continued.

"I am a failed Head of State. I should have paid more attention to the intentions of my immediate subordinates. I should have been more cautious. I bear the shame of thrusting some members of my family into poverty and my country into chaos. That's why I want to be regarded as an average citizen rather than a former privileged and respected leader. It's best that I don't go into the details of my rise and fall or dwell on my failures, and it's best that I don't have to answer to those who might know of my downfall."

Pacing ceased, Mr. Nu sat down, took a deep breath and continued, "When I was young, my parents taught me that it was disrespectful to evade a direct question. So, if a doctor asks about my status before I came to this country, I answer that I had been Head of State before I left my country."

I was thankful to have a detailed answer to my question and gave assurance that his confidences would be honored.

A referral for an imaging stress test was in order. When the results were markedly abnormal, a consultation was requested. The consulting physician was a coronary angiographer with a reputation for being an extraordinary technician which placed him among the elite in his specialty of interventional cardiology. After he performed a complex angioplasty, Mr. Nu did well.

About a month later, I spotted the consulting doctor in the lunch room. I sat beside him, mentioned that our mutual patient continued to be asymptomatic and casually asked if he had learned anything about our patient during his consultation, during lulls of the angioplasty procedure or during their other conversations.

His face went blank. There was a long pause.

"Of course I learned about him," he answered, a bit prickly.

And then he added, "He's an immigrant."

Once I Was Strong

"Now I am weak, but once I was strong."

Those were his first words. He then extended his right hand and in a soft voice uttered, "My name is Anthony."

What stood before me was a wavering body supported by a cane; a short, slight man whose dominant descriptives were "breathless, and wheezing." I guided him to a chair for fear that he might topple. There he sat for a while, seeking relief from the torment of air hunger. He leaned back in the chair and seemed oblivious to his attire that consisted of a crumpled, blue sports jacket and a too-short pair of wrinkled grey pants that exposed swollen ankles above feet stuffed into loosely laced sneakers. He seemed to be a broken man.

His was a common story of progressive-difficulty breathing. A symptom attributed in error to pulmonary problems, rather than to congestive heart failure. The proper diagnosis was made so late that heart power could not be restored.

Anthony Bardolino immigrated to this country from Italy in 1954 at the age of 55. He was now 75, tottering and gasping for breath that flowed to and from congested lungs best described as a set of overworked bellows. Armed with a sketchy referral from the primary doctor prior to meeting with Anthony, I decided to see him at the hospital's out-patient department, anticipating that I might have to send him directly to the emergency department for admission.

Anthony was unaccompanied. The 30-yard walk from the elevator to the waiting area had been exhausting. When his breathing slowed, I explored his past medical history, and then went on to his social history. Anthony came to the United States at age 55. His close relatives were casualties of WWII—all had died from battle wounds, unknown causes or disease. He was sponsored by a church in the Italian enclave of the city, and had been guaranteed work in a bakery. Ten years ago, he became a fractional owner of a small restaurant that specialized in Northern Italian Food. He was close with his employees. They were a substitute for his lost family.

I asked, "What was life like in Italy before you came to this country?"

Between faster than normal respirations, he answered with a few well-chosen words in an expressionless soft monotone, "I swam in my youth.... Post-war construction until an arm injury...then a cook.... Now I am weak, but then I was strong."

While Anthony was changing into an examining gown behind a curtain that separated us, I asked, "What did you mean when you said that you swam as a young man?"

No answer. After a long pause, I persisted.

"Did you swim in the ocean?"

"No, too dangerous."

"Did you swim in a lake?"

"No, too dangerous."

"Did you swim in a river?"

"No, too dangerous."

"Then, did you swim in a swimming pool?"

"Yes."

After Anthony had changed into a gown, he opened the curtain. I was encouraged by his last, one-word, positive response and was determined to continue this line of questioning into Anthony's past and to learn why he was guarding the activities of youth.

"Did you swim for exercise or competitively?"

"Competitively"

"Did you swim for your college?

"Yes"

"Did you swim for your country?"

"Yes"

"Were you an Olympian?"

"Yes"

"Were you a medalist?"

"Yes. Silver."

He got silver, whereas I just struck gold! I told Anthony that I followed many Olympics, that I had been in Rome in 1960 when that city prepared to host the XVII Olympiad. I mentioned that my favorite movie was *Chariots of Fire* and asked, "Have you ever seen it?"

His answer was punctuated by frequent pauses, caused by shortness of breath.

"Yes...many times.... Those were my Olympics."

I remained silent. Anthony's eyes were now bright and flashing about, a smile now animated his face, and he held his head high.

Anthony continued, "...and in those 1928 Olympics...I met your Johnny Weissmuller."

I thought to myself, Wow! An Olympian. Second best in the world in a swimming event, and never volunteered a word about it. Why?

So I asked, and was stunned by his answer.

"I am old, feeble, diminished, and weak.... That is how I am...and how I am perceived... I labor to speak slowly... Doctors are impatient.... You are the first to ask me about days gone by...when I was strong."

At the conclusion of the exam, Anthony insisted on returning to the comfort of his home, his restaurant and his substitute family, rather than be hospitalized. After he agreed to home visits by a nurse, I eliminated some of the medication, adjusted others and added a couple.

The greatest benefit of the consultation was having Anthony's dignity and pride restored. I know that, because he left a different man than when he entered, his right index finger pointed to a small pin attached to the left lapel of his crumpled, blue sports jacket.

"Ten years ago...the Olympic Committee gave this to me...and all surviving athletes who had earned a medal."

We parted while Anthony was still living in the moment when he was the second fastest-swimmer in the world.

The Man of Mystery

When a trainee botched a diagnosis during a case presentation, one of my professors would say, "There are no mysterious illnesses, only mysterious doctors."

In time I learned that there is a corollary.

"There are no mysterious illnesses, only mysterious patients."

*

A 35-year-old visitor from London had been admitted to the Coronary Care Unit (CCU) with chest pain and wished to be treated by a senior cardiologist. So that night I promptly left home for the hospital.

Upon entering the patient's room, I glanced at the cardiac monitor. The blood pressure, heart rate, heart rhythm and respiratory rate were normal. An intravenous line was attached far above his blanket-covered left wrist and an automated blood-pressure cuff encircled his right upper arm. I introduced myself to Charles Kingsley. He was propped up on two pillows. His jet-black hair was parted on the right, so I made a mental note that he was left handed. He had narrow-set non-sinister eyes, a nose slightly crooked—perhaps broken in the past—and a broad smile that displayed shining, straight teeth. Charles looked concerned. The nurses who had cared for him prior to my arrival would later tell me that, overall, Charles was good looking, and appeared to be a "ladies' man."

Our patient was passing through Boston on business. His long flight from London's Heathrow Airport had landed past sundown at Logan International Airport, where he experienced chest pain and an ambulance delivered him to the hospital.

Charles recounted a past history of ischemic coronary heart disease, three years prior. His heart muscle was oxygen starved because its fuel lines were narrowed by fatty deposits that caused chest pain and a minor heart attack. A change in lifestyle and low-dose aspirin had totally eliminated symptoms of heart trouble. Charles told me that the record could be obtained from Dr.

Brian Dowling, an attending cardiac specialist at the Institute of Cardiology at the National Heart Hospital, London.

His only other encounter with the medical establishment was a hiatus-hernia repair for intolerable heartburn. An ugly scar curved around Charles' left chest from back to front, or front to back depending on your vantage point.

With profound pride, Charles spoke of his work for an international consulting firm based in Washington, D.C. He had been stationed in London for four years and had returned to the States to report on the results of exhaustive negotiations with leaders of our North Atlantic Treaty Organization (NATO); the subject—radar installations. Before returning to Washington, he needed to review the latest classified advanced-radar specifications from specialists at the US Department of Defense research program at Massachusetts Institute of Technology's Lincoln Laboratory.

I tried to reassure Charles by explaining that there was no firm evidence of heart damage on the admission electrocardiogram; that there are times that severe chest pain might be from a non-cardiac cause and that several days would be required to assess the significance of the episode. Charles listened attentively.

His dark eyes brightened as he stared at me; then he said, "Doctor, I have confidence in your management. I feel secure here. The morphine I received earlier makes me sleepy. I will have a good night."

I asked, "Do you want me to notify anyone that you are here and currently comfortable; perhaps a relative or your employer?"

"No, Doctor. No need to worry my only remaining kin in Albany, New York. I'd rather that my business associates not know about this yet, or anyone else," he replied.

"Sure. I'll see you in the morning."

The next day, I checked the blood tests before visiting Charles. There were no elevations in the cardiac enzymes that are tell-tale markers of heart damage. When a heart cell dies, its membranous envelope ruptures and its contents are released into the fluids that surround the tissues, then on to the blood stream. In the event of damage, one of the unique cardiac-specific enzymes would be expected to be elevated during the first 24 hours and other cardiac-specific enzymes should elevate thereafter.

Charles was in good spirits after a sound sleep and pain-free morning. He seemed pleased with the preliminary report and the prospect of soon being liberated from bed. All was going well. The plan was routine and straightforward. If only the course could have remained that way!

Some of the staff resident-trainee physicians were consumed with interest in the medical and social aspects of Charles' case. They asked if I knew any more than they about the man. He wasn't a medical curiosity, but what was he? Was he a consultant for the defense department? He had mentioned generic radar to me. To others he mentioned radar, Airborne Warning and Control Systems, intercontinental missiles and having been to politically troubled spots throughout the world. Some of the staff speculated that Charles worked for our government's Central Intelligence Agency (CIA). That speculation became a rumor that morphed into a soft fact which elevated Charles to celebrity status.

That late evening, the CCU rang up my home phone. Charles was having ongoing chest pain that had been unresponsive to three nitroglycerin tablets. Vital signs were stable, but the electrocardiogram had nonspecific changes.

"Damn it, we're back at square one," I said, and I then added, "You had better administer morphine."

Charles remained anxious and unstable for two days. His agonizing chest pains were only relieved by intermittent intravenous morphine.

He asked how I was going to prevent the heart pains, and about an alternative to narcotics for pain relief. I generalized that I hoped we could eliminate the pains with a variety of medications and added that I hoped he could soon start to slowly resume normal activities.

"That might be difficult, Doctor. My work entails a hectic lifestyle with travel and tension."

I drew closer to his bedside and purposely looked straight down at him.

"Exactly what is involved in your work?" I asked.

"Consulting."

"You have been in the Coronary Care Unit four days; do you want to contact your employer? We can bring you a phone."

"No need. Not yet. They often don't hear from me for extended periods of time."

The CCU personnel were correct. Charles was vague and evasive when it came to his work or himself.

I was without a confirmed diagnosis. I did not have a cohesive story for heart pain. Indeed, there was subjective chest discomfort, but there wasn't simultaneous concurrent objective evidence, such as the usual rise in blood pressure and heart rate, or abnormal heart sounds that accompany heart pain. There was absence of blood markers of heart damage, and there were only nonspecific electrocardiographic changes that varied with and without symptoms.

While still standing by the bedside I asked myself if I had previously missed the physical signs of a dissecting aneurysm of the aorta. Best practice should be to check again to eliminate dissection from the differential problem list. A quick test for dissecting aortic aneurysm consists of listening for an aortic-valve heart murmur and taking the blood pressure in both the arms and legs in search of a significant difference in each pairing. Charles objected to taking the blood pressure in the left arm because that might disturb the intravenous line. In retrospect, Charles had either purposefully protected his left arm or naturally did everything with his right hand. I settled for comparing the palpable pulses of the right and left radial wrist arteries. They were equal. No evidence of an aortic dissection. When I was through, he quickly replaced his left hand under the bed sheets. Too late, for I had noticed barely perceptible parallel pale scars about two inches above the inner wrist.

When I asked about the scars, without hesitation, the answer was, "The result of a childhood accident when I lived in Albany, New York. While playing, I crashed my hand against a glass window pane that broke and cut me. Blood spurted everywhere. Luckily someone temporarily stopped the flow with a tourniquet until the doctors fixed it. That event was almost totally lost in memory."

That history was a revelation. The day before, I learned that the record keepers from the National Heart Hospital in London were diligently trying to locate his medical record. Without it, I could not confirm the story of past coronary disease. But why should I doubt it? My inner voice told me to just be patient, but my inner voice also asked, "Why had Charles been hiding the scars?"

I stepped back about 10 feet from the bedside.

"I want to do a simple eye test. Open both eyes and point to the tip of my nose. You can point with your right index finger. Got it? Okay. Now close your right eye. Did your finger move off target?"

Charles answered "No."

"Now open both eyes and close your left eye. Did your finger move off target?"

Charles answered with a head nod to indicate "Yes."

I was reassured that his eyes were fine and I started to leave.

"Before you go, Doctor, I don't want to become a drug addict. Can you find a substitute for the morphine?

"We'll switch to a non-addicting pain killer."

"What if the medical program doesn't work?"

My parting words were, "I'll cross that bridge if we get to it."

The doctors' lounge was close by. While sipping a coffee, I wondered why Charles was hiding, and not using, his left hand when he was most likely left handed. He sighted with his left eye and parted his hair in the same manner as most lefties. By the time I had drained my cup, I wondered if those scars had been self-inflicted.

Fortunately chest pain improved. It was less frequent, less intense and less prolonged. Relief was now obtained with one nitroglycerine tablet. Vital signs remained normal, and the electrocardiograms were unchanged during pain. My patient was on the mend after five days in the CCU. Perhaps he would have an equal portion of good luck during this event as he had after his heart attack three years ago.

The CCU was full, which was a frequent occurrence considering the bounty of acute illness that our hospital attracted. Charles had occupied a bed for five days because of an uncertain diagnosis and my taking the safest course by considering a worst-case scenario. At the moment he was the most stable of the eleven patients in the unit. It was time for transfer to a general-medical floor. He should understand that there must be a bed available to receive an acutely ill patient, just as there had been a bed available to receive him in his moment of need.

"Doctor, I need a private room when I leave here."

"I'll try to arrange that, but be aware that most medical insurers only cover a semi-private room. You will be responsible for the difference."

"Doctor, I need the privacy. I'm feeling better and will be making some phone calls. The differential cost is unimportant. Get me the best room."

What was the need for privacy? Maybe he will call his superiors and discuss issues of national security. Maybe he actually works for the CIA. My inner voice beckoned, "Hey—stop it. Leave all intrigue to those who worry about such things."

The transfer went smoothly. Mild chest pains occurred each day at unpredictable times. Medications were adjusted. Walking about did not aggravate chest pains. Progress at last.

Transfer from the CCU necessitated a new team of nurses and medical trainees. There was a new wave of speculation and intrigue. Was there a link to a private enterprise, a governmental agency—if so, which government, an international arms dealer, organized crime? Some believed we were treating an assassin because a nurse overheard the word "eliminate" during a hushed phone conversation.

The next day we greeted each other with the usual amenities, the usual questions and the customary routine of taking the blood pressure, palpating the pulses, listening to the heart and lungs and examining the abdomen. All was in order.

Even as a senior physician, I learned to expect the unusual, and so it was this day.

"Doctor, when am I going to have my heart catheterization?"

"What heart catheterization?"

"Isn't that what you have to do when a patient's heart pains persist?"

"Yes, at times, but what do you know about heart catheterization? We never discussed it."

He shot back, "Your intern, Doctor Matthews, and I were talking." Charles continued by starting cautiously, proceeding incrementally and ending by speaking with increasing volume and emotion, "I want to have the catheterization. I will agree to it. I will sign the release. I demand it."

Never before had a patient demanded such a test. It is necessary to properly prepare each patient for a diagnostic catheterization. It might lead to a coronary intervention, perhaps the need for coronary surgery. The test cannot be discussed in isolation of its implications and its risks. Its results provide both direction and imperatives for management—continued medical treatment or an intervention. Discussions are painstakingly prepared and are purposefully slow and deliberate.

I asked Charles what he knew about heart catheterization and coronary angiography. In answer to my inquiry, this mystery man expounded on the indications for the procedure, its technical aspects and its complications. The monologue was so thorough and in depth, I thought that we should change places.

"Charles, when did you learn so much? Were there discussions during your convalescence three years ago?"

"No, I discussed it with Dr. Matthews, the intern on your team."

I thought to myself, "Damn Mathews, what is he trying to do. I don't delegate these matters to others."

"You are well informed, but the timing is wrong. You are improving. If you continue to improve, you can rehabilitate wherever you wish—in Boston, Maryland, New York, D.C. or elsewhere. If you falter in your progress, or if you can't function normally—then and only then should we proceed with a heart study. Now is not the time."

Charles resisted, but agreed to wait a little longer. As soon as I had that concession, I beat a retreat. What a way to start the day, a morning that coupled an irresponsible intern and a nervous, demanding patient. Dr. Matthews, in a masterful understatement, denied any more than a casual reference to a heart catheterization.

Expect the unexpected. Progress was moving in the right direction by objective measurements, but subjective response to discomfort was exaggerated pain. Perhaps hypnotic suggestion might diminish his pain. I'd witnessed its benefits in the past.

I was surprised when Dr. Gregory Jay's watch-dog secretary put my telephone call directly through to him. I explained the problem. He was a practicing board-certified psychiatrist who also specialized as a therapeutic hypnotist. He agreed to help lessen the intensity, or eliminate pain through post-hypnotic suggestion. Charles wanted no part of hypnosis when it was presented to him. I explained that he had nothing to lose and everything to gain. Unlike heart catheterization, there was no risk. He finally said that he would give it a try.

What collateral secrets would be revealed this morning while under hypnosis? Perhaps we would learn something helpful, something about his past or about his present circumstances. I could not wait for the results.

Finally, Gregory Jay called. "A total failure. Charles would not be hypnotized. It was clear that he had resisted, was closed, defensive, untrusting and never permitted the proper ambience that allows a patient and hypnotist to have a successful outcome."

The hypnotist tactfully accepted full blame for the failed session, apologized to Charles and promised to make amends by trying again later that day. Charles graciously agreed.

My hospital beeper signaled that the Admissions Office wanted a return call. I was soon saying, "What do you mean nothing checks out!" None of Charles' medical-insurance policies could be verified. Was there a fault in the search? The Admissions Office reported their preliminary findings and would continue the chase.

Whoever said that being a medical doctor would be easy? I formulated my next plan during a boring administrative meeting, and then went to find his room vacant. Poor timing—he was away with Dr. Jay. I scanned the room for a clue. My eyes darted about until they rested upon a partially opened bedside table drawer. Therein lay the bent corner of a brown leather wallet. Did it hold secrets like name, rank and serial number? My conscience told me that it should remain undisturbed. The doctor-patient relationship is sacrosanct. Yet an overpowering force directed my right hand to extract the wallet in search of any clues within its wrinkled leather folds; and confounding information there was. The top line of an identification card read, Name: Fredrick Angel. The next line, Address: Everett, MA. The only other demographic information was a plastic-coated, inner-city hospital photo I.D. card issued to patient Edward Scott. The head-shot photo was Charles Kingsley. I jotted down the patient-identification number, replaced the wallet and stealthily departed.

"Record room please." Silence. "I am a doctor with an unusual urgent request. I am caring for a trauma patient with amnesia. All I have is a name and your hospital's patient identification number. Would you look up the patient's record and tell me his diagnosis? Yes, I'll speak to your supervisor."

The request was repeated. Eventually I heard a voice with an odd dialect emanate from the phone against my ear: "Attempted Suicide and Sociopathic Personality."

I replied, "Thank you for your help. Good day."

I kept repeating the diagnosis out loud: "Sociopathic Personality. Sociopathic Personality." With each repetition, the puzzle became clearer until all the pieces fit. Charles had Munchausen's Syndrome, named after Baron Munchausen who was a teller of tall tales. Fabricators enjoy an enormous sense of self-satisfaction and importance when they deceive the medical establishment. When a fully committed Munchausen zealot presents with feigned or self-induced symptoms or signs such as pain, bleeding, fever, medication-induced altered body function and any number of other signs and symptoms—the fraud might even end with surgery. The deception is the narcotic-like endorphin high, the thrill. Charles had studied hard to present a credible medical deception. Who knows if his left chest scar was the result of a previous faux medical complaint?

The American Medical Association had a Munchausen Register of deceivers' names and their presenting complaints. The names Charles Kingsley, Fredrick Angel and Edward Scott did not appear. Damn it. There was a sick region within Charles' brain that exploited victims for his pleasure. He occupied a bed in a critical unit that could have been used by others in true need; he deceived members of a health-delivery team who were earnestly trying to help him; and he might have worn me down and injured himself by insisting on an unnecessary coronary angiogram that could lead to a complication.

Charles' ultimate goal was to achieve and sustain the thrill of deceit. He was not after the thrill of narcotics; addiction would have been too high a price. Yet his psychologically unbalanced mind could accept unnecessary procedures and worthless surgery to prove his sense of superiority by exposing the fallibility of expert medical opinion. While administrators were suspicious, I had not heeded their concern.

My dark thoughts were interrupted by a beeper page from Dr. Jay. The second session was as useless as the first. When I informed Dr. Gregory Jay that Charles was a total fraud, he was not surprised.

"Don't ask me how I found out. What's the best way to deal with him?"

I believed that was a reasonable question to a psychiatrist about a patient with a troubled mind.

"Get rid of him. He's a hopeless case. If you confront him, he will deny all. If you press him, he will walk out of the hospital. I know. I've had experience with these types."

So I decided to discharge Charles the next morning. The deceiver was seated eating hot cereal when I arrived. As soon as he placed his spoon on the breakfast tray I told him that he had received maximal hospital benefits and would be discharged.

"But, Doctor, I am still having angina. Neither the medicines nor the hypnotist have eliminated my chest pains. Don't you think I deserve heart catheterization to resolve my problem?"

"No, the indications for catheterization are not clear enough. Let's see how you do during the next few weeks. Call my office for an appointment in one week. You can stay at a nearby hotel or at a friend's house."

I concluded by handing Charles a prescription for a common, mild pain medication. He appeared to be in deep thought as he sat on the edge of his bed with vacant sunken eyes and lips locked together. Finally he spoke.

"You make the discharge arrangements. I'll make a few calls and leave after lunch."

I breathed a sigh of relief. That was easier than I thought.

He drank from his coffee cup, replaced it on his tray, gathered himself to stand upright and asked,

"Doctor, how much will you charge for your services?"

"Don't concern yourself about that, I'll bill your insurance." I answered while thinking—why is he prolonging this farce?

"You don't understand, Doctor. I don't want my employer to know about my heart condition. I intend to pay you and the hospital directly."

This was too much. The fabricator was mounting another deception. He walked to the narrow clothes closet, reached in, and returned with a checkbook in hand. I started my day intending to simply let Charles walk out of the hospital. He had succeeded in his murky mission and I had learned a valuable lesson. But now he was adding insult to injury. I couldn't passively let him have another laugh, the last laugh. My response was spontaneous and a work in progress.

"Your case has been a challenge. We have worked hard at a solution. You have been through a difficult time. I don't know how much we have helped you. You have been a model type of patient, as good as I have ever seen. Charles, you have taught me a lot—you don't owe me anything. I don't want to charge you a red cent."

"Doctor, Doctor, why not?"

I moved towards the imposter, and before abruptly pivoting to leave the room, whispered an answer to his question.

"Because, I don't have a real license. I'm not a real doctor."

CHAPTER THREE
Spirituality and Belief

Introduction

Belief about external powers that may or may not influence events and outcomes are personal. In general, it is "politically incorrect" and a breach of etiquette to inquire. Yet, in a doctor-patient relationship, that knowledge is important to define a course of action or inaction. A patient's beliefs, spiritual or otherwise, can determine in whom, what or where the individual finds hope for a satisfactory outcome during a mid-life crisis, an illness or an end-of-life decision.

I will touch on some of the issues in this trio of stories and return to the importance of spirituality and belief at a later time.

Denial

The two-way radio that connects the hospital emergency unit and the city emergency-medical services rang, followed by a crackling transmission that an ambulance was en route with a man in cardiac arrest; expected arrival time—five minutes. The dying patient's name was Anthony Simonetti. The emergency-medical-technician's voice abruptly stopped, leaving the wail of a siren before the sign-off.

Anthony, or Tony, was well known to the hospital. He had a charmed life. Frequent cardiac decompensations had always resolved, even though his heart as "a mechanical pump was a structural disaster." Rumor had it that Tony's heart was kept in working order by a mysterious occult force. How else could a heart function that had muscle damage, leaking valves, clogged fuel lines and a faulty electrical system?

I was assigned the Simonetti case. I would be the doctor of record. When Tony arrived, he would be rushed into a room that was being prepared to receive him.

I'd never met the man but reflected on what little knowledge I had absorbed during frequent presentations of Tony and his heart problems at cardiac conferences.

At age 80, Tony had a strong mind and a weak body supported by a spine that caused him to resemble a punctuation comma when viewed from the side. Kyphosis is the medical term for his extreme forward-arching posture caused in part from a "broken back" incurred when he fell two stories off a scaffold at a construction job. Luckily his broken legs and backbone healed, but at a cost. Tony was permanently disabled at age 51, could no longer work and could be immediately recognized in his Italian enclave as he slowly shuffled along, arched at the waist with head and neck almost parallel to the ground and stabilized from falling forward by two short walking sticks powered with hands and arms strengthened by decades of lugging and laying bricks.

The wheeled stretcher raced towards its destination surrounded by a blur of personnel. One was a heavy-set man trying to perform rapid, chest-cardiac compressions that should transmit enough force to squeeze blood from the heart into the central circulation. Off with Tony's shirt and undershirt and then on with a cardiac monitor, wall oxygen and secure intravenous lines. The heart-rhythm monitor revealed the worst kind of cardiac arrest—a flat line that represented total absence of any electric forces.

Transmitted chest-to-heart compressions are effective if the heart can be compressed between the breast bone and spine. The back must be flattened against a hard surface, otherwise the effort is an exercise in futility. The back of Tony's chest could not flatten. It was more like a rocker rung on a rocking chair. The total effort during the hectic trip from home to hospital was in vain. Tony was dead on arrival. All life signs were absent. The body was cool, the skin mottled, pale and blue; there were no spontaneous respirations; the pupils were dilated and unresponsive to light; there was no heart beat or pulse and no cardiac electrical activity.

Tony was dead. All personnel agreed. So he was pronounced. The family must be notified.

Someone asked, "Are any members present and waiting for a report?"

A voice answered, "Yes, his daughter Rose is waiting."

The next string of directives was my call: "Place Rose in a private family room. Clean up this treatment room. Cover the body from the neck down, and make Tony look as presentable as possible while I speak to his daughter."

From a distance, Rose appeared to be older than her 50 years; she was thin and short in stature; her fingers drumming on the arm of her chair. As I entered the room, she looked at me with inquiring penetrating eyes that were tear-streaked with mascara. Rose stood, then sat in response to my hand signal. I introduced myself. When she asked, I answered that her father died after the first responders did all they could to save him. We continued the effort but his lifeless body would not revive. He died before arriving at the hospital.

Rose went limp. "That can't be. Every time I got him here, he lived to come home. I'm supposed to get him here and you're supposed to get him better. I got him here. Dead? I don't believe you. Let me see for myself."

We went to the treatment room. Her father's head and shoulders were propped up on several pillows with closed eyes towards us as we entered.

Rose settled into a chair, face to face with her father, seeking and finding a lifeless powerless hand. I excused myself to grant her a few solemn private moments with her father. When I returned, she said in a whisper that I was mistaken.

"He is alive—not dead."

"But Rose, there are no signs of life. Look, he isn't even breathing."

She persisted in a whisper, "Yes he is. I've been watching. It's barely perceptible."

Even though there was an urgent need to clear this room for someone in the crowd of waiting patients, I instinctively knew that Rose and her denial of death could not be rushed.

My patient was dead, yet the doctor-patient relationship extends to the patient's entire family. So I asked about the family and how Rose and her father got along.

She told me that her father and mother met in this country. She was the middle child of seven. Two had died young; an older brother from meningitis and a younger sister from viral myocarditis. The oldest brother became a Priest and the oldest sister a Nun. The younger sisters respectively became a school teacher and a nurse before they married. Eventually, all were assigned or voluntarily moved to remote areas. When her mother was killed in an accident, Rose withdrew from nursing school to look after the household which consisted of her younger sisters and also her father who became disabled four years later.

She continued her story while intermittently squeezing her father's hand and caressing the forehead of his blood-drained, blue-lipped pale face.

For the past 30 years she had cared for Tony. He was the center of her universe. They lived in a walk-up apartment. The staircase was narrow with several right-angled turns. For many years Tony would grasp the railing and slowly pull himself up several steps with his powerful hands, then sit on a step to rest before repeating the performance. Going down the staircase was more complicated. Tony would grasp the rail and descend backwards while

Rose stood behind him to guide his legs and to act as a barrier if he fell toward her.

Without fail, they attended nearby Saint Joseph's Church on Sundays and holy days.

This evening, while knitting a sweater, Rose became alarmed by gurgling sounds coming from her father's room. When she investigated, he was upright in his chair with labored breathing oblivious to her or the television that blared before him. Pink foam dribbled from his mouth down his chin. Rose ran to the phone, called 911. After what seemed like a lifetime, the first responders arrived.

Becoming more animated, her words ran together without pause, and her arms waved about as she described the crisis.

In vivid memory, Rose recalled that the emergency crew administered oxygen, barked words like "pulmonary edema" and "morphine" and carried her father down the stairs on a kitchen chair. She followed and wouldn't let the ambulance driver leave without taking her with him. In this business, a life is measured in minutes so, rather than argue, the driver reluctantly agreed. She jumped in and sat buckled in the front passenger seat. As they departed from the house, above the wail of the siren, she heard from behind: "Heart slowing," then, "Cardiac arrest." During the hectic race to the hospital, and while waiting in the Emergency Unit, she clutched her rosary beads and prayed and prayed and prayed.

Rose ended with, "He is alive. He is central to my life."

I thought to myself, "That's the master key. His death would be her death. How can she be convinced that he is dead and she is alive?"

I hesitated a long moment and asked if she wanted to call any of her siblings or close friends. She could use the phone in our private family conference room.

"No." She would remain with her father and protect him from harm.

I hesitated, and then ventured, "His appearance is ghastly. Shouldn't we call a Priest?"

She agreed, while admonishing herself for not taking the initiative. She would remain by her ghost-like father's side while I made the arrangements.

I called the parish that services our Catholic patients in their time of need. Their mission is to serve the ill and needy. Their members are wonderful, tactful and always helpful in alleviating anguish. After Father Dominic arrived, I explained the extraordinary circumstances that he would encounter when I would formally introduce him to Rose and Anthony Simonetti. I did just that, and then slowly drifted over to the farthest corner of the room to become a silent observer.

The priest and Rose briefly conversed in low tones. Father Dominic then invoked some prayers in Latin for the dying or the dead, or both. He then drew a cross on Tony's forehead with his finger. He looked directly at Rose. When their eyes locked, he calmly said, "Your father lives. He has joined your mother, brother, and sister in Heaven. Now it is time for me to take you home." With one hand he beckoned Rose to rise from her chair; with the other he simultaneously drew the blanket over Tony's head. They nodded and left in silence.

I was transfixed. Me, dressed in a long white laboratory coat and a black-tubed stethoscope hanging about my neck. He, completely dressed in black except for a white collar. She, not trusting my pronouncements while having absolute faith and trust in the authority that he represented.

I watched them disappear into the blackness of the night and hoped that Rose would rise from the near dead to find a cause, a purpose, to dedicate her days. To live again.

May God Guide Me

Her mind was clear as a proverbial bell, but it resided in an old body and was being called upon to make a crucial decision. At age 85, Sophie Eisen was at a crossroads. Her facial wrinkles, a broad smile, and alert dark eyes were the markers of kindly wisdom. The source of the problem was deep within her chest. Her heart was failing under the continuous strain of progressive narrowing of the aortic valve. Her aortic stenosis had already been addressed twice with partial opening of the critically narrowed valve by a procedure called catheter balloon dilatation or aortic balloon valvuloplasty. Debilitating limited-exercise tolerance, breathlessness and fluid retention from congestive heart failure had temporarily improved after each procedure but had predictably recurred within a year. Once again, familiar unwanted symptoms had emerged. Fortunately, other troubles associated with critical aortic stenosis had not, such as life-threatening arrhythmias, fainting spells and chest pain.

The chronology was the late 1980s. It was a time when heart surgery had matured and individual hospital outcomes and individual heart surgeon's results were not yet public information. It was a time when surgeons were willing to perform high-risk operations to save lives, rather than decline high-risk operations to protect their own reputations. The place was a major medical center. Sophie's prognosis was poor. Her life hung on a thin thread. Without heart-valve replacement, she would soon die. Aortic valve replacement in the elderly is a major undertaking. Over time, the age of the surgically qualified "elderly" increased from sexagenarians to octogenarians. Dr. Jerome, a highly skilled surgeon had twice before passed judgment and still believed that Sophie was a reasonable, yet high, surgical risk. Any further physical deterioration would exclude a surgical intervention.

Sophie's position had been firm. She was opposed to open-chest, heart-valve replacement. She accepted the far-less invasive, balloon catheter stretching open of her valve. Because of diminishing returns with the balloon procedure, direct heart-valve replacement was the only remaining intervention. A scary possibility, because that procedure had many associated adversities including death, stroke and severe infection, to name a few.

Guided by life-long religious precepts, Sophie was outwardly and inwardly a deist, strengthened by her teachings, prayers and faith. She was in the twilight of her life. It had been a good life. She was a widow, but her husband lived on in her memory and in her kind heart. She was blessed with children and grandchildren. Her family provided a strong support system at all times. Sophie believed that death was inevitable and had hopes that she could live out her remaining days, or months, in comfort. On the other hand, her teaching had always been to choose a painful life in opposition to death.

While she was recovering her strength in the hospital, I had many a lengthy discussion with Sophie about the pros and cons of the surgical option. She displayed unusual wisdom in not wanting her family's guidance on the matter. She would decide what to do. Her family should not have self-recrimination if the outcome of surgery was disastrous, or if she died while firmly opposed to having surgery. She would think on the matter and come to a decision. Would she be a courageous patient that placed herself in the hands of a courageous surgeon?

The days passed without a decision as Sophie prayed for guidance. As we waited, tentative preparations were being made for surgery in case Sophie agreed. Yet there was no sign from on high and no decision.

Finally: "I think I have the answer, but I am still struggling with the question. I will tell you tomorrow."

The next day I cautiously asked, "Have you decided?"

"Yes, I will leave it up to God."

"Then you don't want surgery and you will let the illness run its natural course."

"Oh, no." she protested, "I want the surgery, and may God guide Dr. Jerome's hands."

Caught Between Two Sciences

As a medical student, I was assigned to a relatively under-supervised surgical service at a major teaching hospital. The interns and a hierarchy of resident trainees made most of the decisions. The doctors were postgraduate, resident, house officers who lived in the hospital and were continuously busy with emergency admissions of medically neglected inhabitants of the surrounding underserved urban community. Preventative medicine seemed to be an anathema. Many patients had addictive habits that ensured ill health and death at an early age. The most culpable were tobacco, alcohol and poor nutrition that either occurred singularly—or more likely in a lethal combination.

I was assigned to a team of four postgraduate trainees who were charged with the task of supervising my introduction to surgical healing. The team was comprised of an intern as well as a junior, senior and chief resident. I was directed to newly admitted patients whose medical problems would be a "teaching moment" for a novice. That is how I met Maxwell Thorton, a learned gentleman whose financial reverses "temporarily" landed him in a nearby rental apartment. His chief complaint was progressive back pain that he stoically tolerated, with an occasional grimace during my meandering extraction of Maxwell's history. At the conclusion of the exercise, he told me, "Just call me, Max."

With the exception of dental visits and an involuntary, World War II, draft-induction, physical examination that he failed because of severe hypertension, Max avoided contact with medical practitioners during his 55-year life. Max sat on the edge of his bed across from me. He was clean shaven, alert, rosy cheeked, balding and expressed well organized thoughts in clearly understandable language. Being from a middle-class background with an elite Ivy League college education, and without obvious psychiatric problems, he was in a distinctly different category than our usual patient population. Max was also a rarity among the overwhelming majority of patients who seek care from the medical establishment—he was a second-generation devout member of the Church of Christ, Scientist.

The onset of the current illness started 18 months earlier. While taking a shower, Max felt an abdominal pulsation beating against the palm of his hand. On further exploration, he could define a painless pulsating mass. Intuitively, he knew that he had an important health problem. In accord with his religious faith, a certified practitioner of Christian Science healing was contacted. They regularly prayed together. When the pulsatile mass enlarged during the latter part of the year, Max became so alarmed that he transferred his care to another Christian Science practitioner. The mass got even larger. When back pains became severe, he sought help at our nearby hospital, and did so against the protestations of the practitioner. Yet Max asked to be prayed for even though he believed that the congregants of his church would cast him out for forsaking Christian Science in favor of medical science.

Our doctors immediately diagnosed the huge pulsatile mass as an abdominal aortic artery aneurysm. That is, a weakening of the wall of the main artery that carries blood-born nutrition and oxygen to the vital organs and tissues below the dividing line that separates the chest from the abdomen. The weak aortic wall distends and expands like a blister that becomes weaker and thinner until it bursts. In man's closed circulatory system, each heartbeat pumps a bolus quantity of blood into the aorta that acts like a wave striking all the sides of its tubular wall. Wave after battering wave ultimately ruptures the aneurysmal wall. Then blood pours out of the circulatory system and death from hemorrhagic shock quickly follows.

The chief resident cautioned me to be ultra-gentle while feeling the surface of the aneurysm during my physical examination. Anything more vigorous might rupture the beast. Another of Max's striking physical findings was rigid pipe-like arteries in the legs.

The frequency of aneurysmal rupture has a direct correlation to size. Max was overdue. His blood pressure was lowered to reduce the internal force of each pulse of blood against the aneurysm's wall, while arrangements were hastily made for surgical resection of the aneurysm and replacement with a fabric graft if Max agreed. The procedure would be complex, hazardous and without assurance of success. Max's life hung in the balance.

"Overwhelmed" would be an understatement of Max's state of mind after he was informed (by the "team" and a consulting senior vascular surgeon) of his life-threatening problem, his prognosis and the required surgical procedure to achieve his physical salvation. He had to think about it; about voluntarily renouncing a life-long heritage of church teachings; about transferring his faith and trust from the church to medical science; about his hope for continued life; about his mortality.

When the team departed, I remained. Max spoke about his options while I listened. Do nothing or submit to high-risk major surgery. He could not ask anyone for advice. No living parent. No siblings. His few church friends were fundamentalists who would shun him. Max was single, independent and still self-sufficient. He would think about it. On morning rounds, the chief resident was optimistic about the operative outcome. Max agreed to have surgery as soon as possible in his race with death; hoping the aneurysm would not explode while final preparations were put in place.

The next day, the chief resident was the lead surgeon assisted by the senior resident. I had barely caught up with them in the recovery room when Max came out of anesthesia. His first conscious words were slurred but distinct.

"Thank God I survived. Thank you all."

"Max, we are so sorry," the surgeon explained. "Your aorta was totally calcified. If we removed the aneurysm, the stitches would not have held the fabric graft to the aorta. They would have torn away. So we left things as they were and simply closed you up. Sorry."

I was stunned. Max became wide eyed and fully alert. His faith and trust in doctors must have been instantly shattered. He was an outcast of his church and no longer had hope of remaining on this earth or entering any other realm.

Max stared at the ceiling for a long moment then closed his moist eyes, silently folded himself into a fetal position and waited to die.

CHAPTER FOUR
Always Ask a Patient about Their Pet

Introduction

Pet animals are cherished members of a nuclear family. A pet is usually aware when someone in their household is ill, and they seem to despair until a reasonable recovery occurs.

Pets brightly illuminate the day of the lonely. Temporary visits to residents of healthcare facilities such as nursing homes or assisted-living facilities seem to improve outcomes.

At times, a pet becomes important glue in the bonding between a patient and doctor. Doctors should grant pets a near-equal status to every other member of a patient's family. In 1926, Francis W. Peabody, a popular educator at Harvard Medical School, when addressing the students on The Care of the Patient, had several important messages for every doctor to keep in mind.

He said,
> …it is equally important for the physician to know the exact character of those [home] surroundings.
>
> The clinical picture involves the patient's surroundings; his works, his relations to his friends, his joys, sorrows, hopes and fears.

And finally,
> …the whole problem of diagnosis and treatment depends on your insight into the patient's character and personal life.

So doctors should always ask a patient about their pet.

A Grateful Patient and a Show Dog

On occasion, a grateful patient names a highly regarded animal after their doctor. A case-in-point was a valuable thoroughbred race horse, "Doctor Fager," named after neurosurgeon Charles Fager who successfully treated the horse's trainer, Charles Nerud. Dr. Fager, the thoroughbred, went on to accumulate winnings in high-stakes races. The stallion won four major titles in 1968 and was named Horse of the Year. I was familiar with the story. Imagine, a super horse named after a physician who had saved a patient's life.

Cardiologists save lives by diagnosing life-threatening conditions, instituting medical treatments or performing interventions. I did all of that, so it was natural for me to occasionally wonder if I would have an animal superstar namesake. Well, it almost came to pass.

I looked after a middle-aged couple from Cape Cod, Massachusetts. Lillian was a vibrant bundle of energy whose son and daughter had left the nest. With time on her hands, she started to raise purebred miniature poodles for show. In a short time her kennel and superior blood-line champion poodles were in demand. What started as a hobby became a stressful full-time occupation. Worry about the dogs, the business and irregular hours all contributed to her high blood pressure and overweight status.

Her husband, Harry, was a swarthy muscular construction contractor. He drank, smoked and swore mightily. Lunch breaks were an occasion for a salami or sausage sandwich and a mug of strong coffee. He had peripheral vascular disease, mild diabetes, a chronic cough and high blood pressure. Unfortunately he was not compliant with medications, diet or other recommendations to modify his unhealthy habits.

The couple's unstable health required relatively frequent visits. Lillian and Harry were seen in sequence on the same day. The summary session was discussed with the couple seated across the desk. They were concerned about each other's health. My wish was that Harry would be concerned about his own health. He always said that he would *try* to do better. He never said, "I will do better." His children constantly sermonized to have Harry reform.

They even set an example by becoming vegetarian, and by giving up alcohol and smoking.

When Lillian lost weight and had adequate sleep, her blood pressure normalized without increasing her medication. With constant "bad health habits," Harry developed a prominent asymptomatic abdominal pulsation that proved to be an aneurysm. I had Dr. Marshall Silver, a skilled vascular surgeon, consult. Harry's surgical correction was an immediate success, but the post-operative recovery was slow. During that two-month period, it seemed that whenever I visited Harry in the hospital or rehabilitation center, Lillian was at his side showing him news clippings of one or another of her miniature poodles that had been named "Best in Show" or that had become a national or international champion. Harry ultimately made a complete recovery. As so often happens after a crisis, he realized the error of his ways, totally reformed and became a zealot advocate for others as he walked the narrow path of recommended good-health habits.

Not long thereafter, Lillian and Harry entered the office for their appointment wearing broad smiles while holding two photographs. On each was an image of a newborn miniature poodle. Lillian explained, in gratitude for her husband's recovery, she had named one Doctor Stafford and the other Doctor Marshall. Wow! I immediately thanked Lillian for her gracious gesture while fantasizing that my namesake would become a grand champion.

I heard no more about my dog during the following year. So, the next year, I placed the photograph of Doctor Stafford in a picture cube and prominently displayed it on my desk whenever Lillian had an appointment. On each occasion, she made no comment.

Finally, at the end of the second year without information about my dog, I lost patience and casually made an inquiry about the dogs. There was such a long silence that I imagined Lillian had gone deaf and mute. She finally offered, "I was hoping you wouldn't ask. Doctor Marshall died and Doctor Stafford ate so much—gained so much weight—I couldn't show him."

Shattered dreams.

Service Dog

Angela was a middle-aged, single parent; the mother of Tiffany, a teenage, autistic daughter. A small mixed-breed dog named Goliath was her daughter's best friend. Life had dealt Angela a difficult hand. She was born into poverty, married young to a husband who soon committed suicide when she was pregnant. Their child had learning and developmental disabilities. Fortunately the state of Rhode Island and the federal government provided a safety net with schooling for special-needs children; health insurance; city-managed, low-income, public housing; and food stamps. The health insurance was critical for child and mother after Angela developed diabetes as well as peripheral vascular and cardiovascular disease at a young age. Yet she always appeared to be optimistic—and when asked, "How are things?"—the answer was invariably, "Just fine." I suspected that she was suffering in silence and would occasionally pry a confession that she was bedeviled by an unanswered question about who would care for her daughter if a calamity were to befall either her aging parents or herself. Angela's concerns mounted after she suffered several small heart attacks heralded by atypical symptoms of nausea. In addition, labile diabetes had resulted in hypoglycemia with near fainting on several occasions.

Her visits became more frequent and her reluctance to share her concerns dissipated after my shepherding her from quicksand to solid ground during several hospitalizations, cardiac rehabilitation and followup visits.

At one office visit, she shared a remarkable story. On two separate occasions, while at home in the evening, she had fainted from a severe hypoglycemic attack and lay on the floor unconscious. She was later told that Goliath raced upstairs to her sleeping daughter and raised an alarm by barking and pulling at the blankets and sheets. Tiffany followed Goliath to her unresponsive mother and dutifully dialed 911 as she had been trained in the event of an emergency. It was amazing that a dog and an autistic child could collaborate as a team to repeatedly save a life. I was certain that Angela's primary physician would also be amazed when he read the dog-and-daughter story that became the centerpiece of my consultation note.

All appeared well until a consultation six months later that was prompted by an electrocardiograph change suggestive of an interval "silent" heart attack. After Angela settled herself in a chair, I asked, "How are things with you, Tiffany and Goliath?" Tiffany was well. But sadly Goliath had been adopted by a family friend because three weeks earlier the city had transferred Angela to an apartment in another low-income development that did not permit pets.

"What! Does your primary doctor know about this?"

"He sure does. He filled out the paperwork for the transfer."

"How could he?" I said in disbelief. "Your dog functions as a service dog."

"What is that?" asked Angela.

I explained that the Disabilities Act of 1990 required housing authorities to permit a tenant with diabetes to retain a dog that was trained to provide a service. Although Goliath had no specific training, in an emergency, his natural instincts triggered the same behavior as a trained dog. He qualified as a service dog and should be reunited with Angela and Tiffany at once. I could not rely on the primary physician, so in Angela's presence, I phoned her housing authority. They agreed to permit Goliath to return. With facts in hand, they had no choice. Angela called her friend who was happy to have Goliath continue to service Angela and to provide emotional support and comfort to Tiffany.

Always ask a patient about their dog, or their equivalent pet!

A Dying Man's Wish Fulfilled

Burt was a square-jawed, tough-looking guy. He was powerful and had a physique that outlined most muscle groups. But appearances are deceiving. Burt was an artist, tough only on himself, demanding excellence in every endeavor.

He had immense talent, went to the Massachusetts College of Art on full scholarship and, after one semester, was advised to concentrate on illustration.

Indeed, illustration was Burt's first love, while jazz music was a close second. He had an encyclopedic memory of musicians and their performances. He spent leisure time listening to jazz recordings or attending live shows at Boston's many clubs. Shrouded in a smoke-filled atmosphere, his sketches of the performers captured their mood and their energy. Burt and his art were noticed.

Eventually, Burt became famous. His illustrated jackets of jazz recordings commanded a high price and were exhibited in galleries and museums.

When we first met, age and illness had taken a heavy toll. Although retired, Burt continued to illustrate for pleasure. Burt had a long-term marriage to his wife, Kathy. The childless couple lived in suburbia. They had a happy home life where they shared their abundant affection for each other and a pet bulldog named Winston.

Burt crossed the threshold to my office because of his injured pride and animus towards his prior cardiologist. I could sympathize with Burt in his belief that he was regarded as a number rather than as a person. After one year, his doctor did not know what inspired Burt, his aspirations, his mission or his goals. During the initial visit, the doctor asked what Burt did prior to retirement; "I painted" he had answered and added some words of explanation. The official record listed the profession as a "house painter," rather than as an "artist." Several requests to correct the record were ignored. Because of double bookings, Burt and Kathy often had to wait 30 to 60 minutes beyond their appointed time to have an abbreviated, hurried visit with the doctor. Kathy believed that Burt had more tests administered and supervised by the cardiologist inside and outside of his office than discussions about the need for, or results of, the tests.

Before our first meeting, advanced coronary disease and its sequel of congestive heart failure forced Burt to spend most of his time confined to home where he and Winston became close companions. For exercise, Burt and Winston would slowly walk up their long sloping driveway to the street two or three times a day. When the walk up became progressively more difficult for Burt, Winston understood, slowed to his master's pace and remained close by.

By default, the task of explaining the prognosis of congestive heart failure fell to me. The five-year survival of chronic congestive heart failure is approximately fifty percent. Burt had already survived four years. With encouragement, Burt dedicated himself to his medical regimen and to enjoying what time remained with Kathy and Winston.

There were continuing mini-crises such as brief hospitalizations and intermittent urgent office appointments arranged by the visiting nurse. During those office visits at the end of the day, I would ask "How's your dog, Winston?" Burt and Kathy would then urge me to come to the adjacent parking garage and see for myself. When I did, Winston always appeared happy, calm, quiet and friendly, with his stub tail wagging away.

Eventually, Burt experienced sudden pulmonary edema and was taken by ambulance to our emergency department. Although medical management cleared the fluid from Burt's lungs, and a coronary angiogram showed no change, the improvement was short-lived. Burt remained in the hospital and continued to fail, despite aggressive medical management. Each day, he begged me to permit visitations from Winston. "Winston won't bother anyone," Burt said. "Here I am in a private room!"

I reluctantly replied, "Hospital rules don't permit visits from pets."

With that, I am sure Burt had second thoughts about the words he had previously directed to me on a catalogue of his works, "From the heart of an artist to a doctor with a heart."

Symptoms of end-stage congestive heart failure are difficult to witness. The shadow of the Grim Reaper was outside Burt's hospital room when I left for a distant medical meeting. Burt died before I returned. On the morning of his death, Kathy was by his side, having spent most of the previous night with him.

When I expressed my condolences to Kathy, I shared my remorse at having been away when Burt died, and his not being able to visit with Winston.

Kathy replied, "Don't worry, he died happy. The night nurse and I took care of that."

Kathy explained that Burt had constantly asked for Winston those last few days. The evening nurse thought that it would be tragic if Burt did not get his dying wish—and nurses know how to get things done. She would be working the night shift the next day and would cast a "blind" eye if Kathy entered Burt's room about 1:00 A.M. So during Burt's last two nights on Earth, Kathy came and left in the wee hours of the morning carrying Winston beneath a blanket. Burt held Winston; they kissed each other and said their goodbyes. A kind-hearted nurse had enabled Burt to die a happy man.

CHAPTER FIVE
Near the End of Life: What Gives Meaning to Life?

Introduction

Most people would have difficulty answering the question: How would you choose to spend what little time remains before you die? Persons confronted with that stark reality have innumerable choices.

Some historical examples follow: ignore the Reaper and make the best of it; don't focus on the negative, only on the positive; die happy.

When Norman Cousins, the editor of the *Saturday Review* was diagnosed with a potentially fatal illness by William M. Hitzig, a prominent cardiologist in New York City, Cousins chose to die happy while viewing humorous movies. He survived and wrote a scholarly anecdotal book about the benefits of "Laugh Therapy."[1] Morrie Schwartz, a college professor with amyotrophic lateral sclerosis, so-called Lou Gehrig's disease, chose to be present at his mock pre-mortem memorial service. He didn't want to miss his friends, family and associates' eulogies.[2]

Other historic choices are more somber. Paul Kalanithi, a young neurosurgeon, and his wife Lucy decided to have a child and he succeeded in writing a book about his struggle with impending death from lung cancer.[3]

Some adults draw upon their "To Do" list. Children with deadly disease are helped by the Make-A-Wish foundation. It fulfills a child's wish that previously had been considered an impossible dream.

Yet others near death desire to accomplish an obligation rather than a dream. In 1912, when Antarctic explorer Robert Scott and several of his comrades knew that they would die on their return trip from the South Pole to their base camp, each had the option of having a quick and painless death by taking an overdose of heroin, or the option to die slowly as honorable Englishmen in pursuit of their mission. They all honored their pledge to their

Queen and their countrymen. In doing so, they chose death by slow starvation and hypothermia.[4]

Some of my patients drew up formal documents that contained elements of knowledge and wisdom to guide descendants on their life journeys. Other unfortunates leave a legacy of remembrance by establishing and attaching their name to a scholarship, structure or cause.

A quartet of patient stories follow. Each patient chose a different course before their fate was sealed.

End Notes

1. Norman Cousins. Anatomy of an Illness 1979. WW Norton & Co Inc. New York, NY
2. Mitch Alborn. Tuesdays With Morrie: An Old Man, a Young Man, and Life's Greatest Lesson 1997. Broadway Books a division of Random House. Inc. New York, NY
3. Paul Kalanithi. When Breath Becomes Air 2016. Random House. New York, NY
4. Robert F. Scott. Tragedy and Triumph. The Journals of Captain R.F. Scott's Last Polar Expedition 1993. Konecky & Konecky. New York, NY

A Patient's Dilemma

Ed was an acquaintance and a colleague on the staff of a community hospital. We met when I directed an on-site, monthly, continuing-medical-education session at his hospital, which was the place where he was admitted after coughing blood. He was transferred to my medical center, and was sequestered behind the closed door of his room. I walked by that barrier for several days; but then one day the door was open, and, as I passed, a voice called out for me to enter. Ed, a 48-year-old Emergency Medicine Specialist, was happy to see me and happy to have someone to talk to.

"I've been lonely. Friends have been reluctant to visit because they know I have terminal cancer. I'm so glad that you came by. Let me tell you what's happened to me."

Ed had a youthful appearance, ruddy cheeks, eyes as blue as Colorado's Big Sky and premature gray hair. He was smart, received degrees at elite universities and served a stint in the US Naval Intelligence Service. His tale was grim and his chance for survival even darker. I saw him age before my eyes as he spun his story of being well, coughing blood and having an X-ray that revealed left-chest obliteration by a large lung tumor that had tell-tale signs of cancer. Ed was a two-pack-a-day cigarette smoker for 30 years, preferring (not-so-lucky) Lucky Strikes—even in the face of the U.S. Surgeon General issuing warnings in 1957 and 1964 that cigarettes caused lung cancer.

The prognosis of lung cancer is dependent on tumor size. It was a hard fact that Ed theoretically had no chance for survival. The Chief of Oncology proposed that my colleague either do nothing, or do everything possible. Everything included chemotherapy, followed by radiotherapy, followed by removal of the left lung.

The choices were to continue to feel well until tumor growth caused major pain that would be alleviated with narcotics before death, or to have chemotherapy and immediate misery that would continue throughout the triad of proposed treatments until the overwhelming predicted statistical outcome was finalized—in death.

Ed told me that he had to think long and hard how to spend his remaining limited time of life. He would "sleep on it." I left and promised to visit again.

The decision was to undergo therapy. Ed was obligated to do so for his nuclear family; for his wife and their two dependent children. In his words, "I have an obligation to move forward for the sake of my young children. It's not about me, it's about my family."

After that, I was a constant visitor during intermittent cycles of chemotherapy. During one visit, he was delirious, was talking nonsense and was burning with fever. Bacterial infection too often complicates chemotherapy. It took several days to lower the high fever, and even longer for Ed to regain his mental equilibrium. Somehow he endured the treatments —the chemotherapy, the radiation and the removal of the tumor-infiltrated lung. Recovery was slow. A shrunken frame expanded with the return of appetite, and a ruddy complexion replaced pallor.

I became officially involved when Ed developed exertional heart pain. He was fine with moderate activity, but chest pain occurred with emotional stress or with any burst of physical activity. There were good days, but the unpredictable bad days permanently prevented his return to work. Otherwise life and living had basically returned to a new normal. Ed enjoyed expansive time to be with his family, and he observed and guided his children's continued growth and development.

After two years with cancer in remission and without evidence of tumors, Ed started to receive calls from doctors asking him to cheer up some unfortunate patient or friend with newly diagnosed advanced cancer. Ed accepted, after an agreement with the patient's doctor to set the stage and the script for a proper introduction.

A common scenario would be for a hospitalized patient to be told that a doctor would come by to visit. Eventually, Ed would enter the room and introduce himself. He would ask the patient to, "Tell me your diagnosis." Then he would ask, "What's the outlook?"

A typical answer might be, "Fifty-fifty."

Then the visiting doctor would say, "That's pretty good. When I had cancer, they told me the outlook was near zero."

The frightened newly-diagnosed patient and the cancer survivor, who now appeared to be the picture of health, would talk about how to get through the treatments.

After each visit, a patient had newfound hope and Ed's mission to help others gave new meaning to his life.

All went well, with the exception of an occasional infection emanating from the residual stump of what had been the natural left-lung bronchial breathing tube. Most episodes were mild, but some were severe with evidence of bacteria in the blood stream (bacteremia).

Cancer prognosis is measured in terms of five-year survival rates. There was no evidence of residual cancer and no major problem for ten years. During that time Ed gave hope to many newly diagnosed cancer victims.

Then, one morning Ed could not be roused from sleep. I was contacted after the problem was diagnosed as metastatic cancer of the brain based on a head scan. I thought, "That seemed strange after being cancer free for 10 years." So, I reviewed the scan with the senior radiologist.

I asked, "What is your diagnosis?"

The radiologist answered, "My first, second, and third diagnoses are metastatic cancer to the brain."

"Could it be anything else?"

"No."

"I know this patient well. How about multiple brain abscesses? This patient has a past history of many infections with bacteremia."

"Really! Hell, no one told me. If that's the case, abscess is a possibility."

So the attending staff was informed and indeed there were multiple brain abscesses. With treatment, Ed was once again restored to health and lived for another 16 years.

But what's the best explanation for his 26-year cancer-free survival? In retrospect, that early, intra-chemotherapy-associated, high-grade fever from infection might have been a godsend by boosting the immune system to immobilize and start to destroy lung-cancer cells.

Although Ed did not die of cancer, he always believed that his days were numbered. During the 26 years after being diagnosed, each day of each year had special purpose. He had a constant presence and positive influence on his children. He lived to see them become solid citizens who would be the pride of any parent. Ed was a compassionate doctor, a committed healer who had great success in his unanticipated voluntary post-cancer mission. He became a "Medical Missionary" who was a motivator of hope for multitudes who were stricken with cancer by encouraging those bewildered souls to look forward to better days.

The Master Watchman

The wizened white-haired man before me spoke softly while seated on his hospital bed.

"D-doctor, I know I don't have l-l-long to l-live, and when I die, I want to be remembered."

Seamus Shannon had a premonition of impending death, as did so many others who experienced a slow decline over several years. Each had abruptly transitioned from physical comfort to a struggle for life during intermittent agonizing crises. Now 89, Seamus had survived heart attacks, heart failure, pneumonia, heart arrhythmias and a minor stroke that resulted in temporary right-arm paralysis but did not further trouble his speech. His stammering and stuttering had been a lifelong affliction.

My teaching hospital encouraged long-term, patient-doctor relationships by assigning individual patients to specific trainees. Early into internship, I cared for Seamus during the first of his several heart attacks. I was his guiding doctor for each of his subsequent hospitalizations and at many out-patient clinic visits. Unfortunately the frequency of hospitalizations and clinic visits were directly related to the downward trajectory of ill health.

The stars were not properly aligned the day that Evelyn Shannon gave birth to Seamus. He was fated to be her first and only child. At an early age his cup of life was destined to be filled with tears.

Who was Seamus before he became chronically ill?

He was a life-long stutterer. Excellent hand-eye coordination was countered by a limp that threw him off stride. The combination of unusual characteristics was fodder for brutal bullying that continued until high school graduation. When the stress of being tormented by classmates was lifted, Seamus' father died in an industrial accident. Evelyn Shannon immediately went to work laundering and cleaning house for anyone who would hire her. There were many church members who helped when they learned of her plight.

It was a difficult time to be fatherless. Seamus had earned his high school diploma in a program that emphasized exposure to the "trades," those practical blue-collar jobs. He excelled in automotive repairs, assembling any apparatus and repairing electrical fixtures. He was adrift without fatherly guidance toward a career, or at least a job. The school's guidance office had job postings as did the local newspaper. After each dreaded interview, a letter eventually arrived with a familiar introduction: "We are sorry to inform you..." Then on a rainy day, en route to the food store with his mother's grocery list in his pocket, an invisible hand turned Seamus' head toward a sign in the window of Goldsmith's Jewelry Store that read, "Help Wanted—Inquire Within." The proprietor needed an unskilled helper to perform general tasks such as running errands, having items mailed at the post office, sweeping the floor and cleaning the display cases. A severe speech stutter wasn't a disqualifier because customer contact was not required. He was hired at a low wage and was proud to have a job at long last.

Errands kept him busy most of the day. During slow periods, he observed Max, the busy, bespectacled, elderly watch repairman at his work. Max came to America from Eastern Europe, established his own jewelry shop, and in his later years gave up his shop, and its headaches, to repair time pieces. His work was his love, for Max was a bachelor. He opened Goldsmith's store each morning and was the last to leave each evening. Seamus quietly observed Max while he restored and repaired complicated time pieces. Brief observation periods became addictive and additive. Minutes added up to hours, hours to weeks, and weeks to months. Over time, the observer learned by example. One day Max gave him a watch that was beyond repair. Seamus deconstructed and rebuilt it a dozen times, then asked Max for a "click screw" from his vast collection of spare parts. With the new screw replacement, the watch was restored to working order.

"Congratulations."

"Th-Th- Thank you, M-Max."

Max was aging, his vision was starting to fail and a slight left-hand tremor had made its presence known. When the diagnosis of early Parkinson's disease was established, Max informed Goldsmith that failing vision and an unsteady hand would soon ruin his ability to work. Max suggested that Seamus become his apprentice. Goldsmith was hesitant until

Max reassured him that Seamus was a quick learner, had a keen eye and very steady hands. And so it was, with Max observing his apprentice and telling him what to do, step by step.

When Max retired, Seamus took over as watchman at Goldsmith's Jewelry Store. He, like Max, never married, had a love for his work, entered the store early each morning to ready it for business and tidied it up after hours each evening.

As the years slipped by, Evelyn Shannon died of natural causes, her only child became a master at his craft, and Goldsmith's Jewelry Store changed ownership the same year that Seamus was forced to retire after his first heart attack at the ripe old age of 85.

The next four years were a misery for Seamus who was back and forth from one residential nursing home, to the hospital, and then back to a different nursing home because his bed had been given to another patient the very day it was vacated. Seamus was lonely, without family or friends. He had prayed for each of his lost friends until there were none left. Now there were no friends left to pray for him.

That was a brief summary of Seamus Shannon's life journey before the moment that he rose up from sitting at his bedside, stood by his bed, took a few steps and settled with a sigh into a chair.

"Like I said, D-Doctor, I know I'm going to d-d-die soon. The worst thing about a long l-l-life on this earth is not to b-be remembered. You know me b-better than anyone else. I want you to remember me."

"Off course I will. How could I ever forget? You are so skilled. I am always awestruck that your old time pieces remain accurate. Don't be gloomy and morbid. You may have more time than you believe. You'll be discharged tomorrow. I'll see you in the morning before you go back to a nursing home."

The next day I arrived on time, but the transporters had arrived earlier and were wheeling my protesting patient on a gurney towards an elevator. We both demanded that the transporters stop, that they step away and that they give us a few moments of privacy.

"Doctor, I meant what I said yesterday. I have n-no one but you. I want you to have this watch rather than have it g-go to the g-grave with me." With that he removed his wrist watch and held it out for me.

"D-Doctor whenever you see or wear it, you will think of me. Remember to wind it every so often so its movement doesn't freeze up."

"I don't need the watch as a reminder. I promise that I will not forget you."

Seamus started to get agitated; his soft voice raised a few decibels, and without a stutter emphatically said, "Life can be strange. You have been my sole support these past years. Don't forget your promise."

With those words, he rose as far as his gurney restraints would permit, thrust the watch into the side pocket of my white jacket, and beckoned to the transporters that he was ready. They swiftly returned and whisked him away as I stood speechless.

That was the last I saw of Seamus Shannon. He died shortly thereafter. The death notice listed his name with "details to follow" that never followed.

I occasionally wear the vintage Longine watch and compulsively wind it. It continues to keep perfect time. Indeed Seamus has not been forgotten. His watch is now considered a family heirloom. It will be handed down from one generation to another along with its provenance.

A promise made is a promise kept.

The Greek Sea Captain

In a gesture of uncertainty, I raised my hands, palms up, shrugged my shoulders, and divined, "A year at most."

I was obligated to answer the question, "Doctor, how long do I have to live?" posed by the old man with the weather-beaten face, crooked mouth and bloodshot brown eyes who sat before me.

Panos Panopolis calmly weighed my verdict. He sighed, and slowly swiveled his head from side to side. His grey beard, straight nose, and high cheek bones appeared to my eyes in alternating right and left profile. He waved his captain's hat, held tightly by gnarled fingers, paused and said,

"I hope you're wrong, but if you're right—that's okay. A year or less might be just enough time."

Panos Panopolis was a retired Greek sea captain. At age 16, he shipped out, became a seaman second class, advanced up the ladder to first class, then to navigator and finally to captain. When the Germans invaded Greece during the Second World War, his ship was docked in New York. Panos established residency in the US and continued to captain ships of many flags to and from the port cities of New York, New Jersey and Philadelphia.

Panos became a naturalized citizen, plied the oceans until a ripe age and was forced to retire when he was no longer "fit for duty" because of heart trouble. His current residence was a retirement home for seamen on the shores of New York Harbor. A perfect location for men of the sea to share their adventures while watching the coming and goings of boats, barges and ships.

Panos had not set foot on Greek soil for 30 years. He was now 80 years old with many medical problems; the most troublesome were heart related. His heart pump had worn out years before and didn't know it. It was deluded with youthful exuberance *except* for a few issues. They were: a severely narrowed aortic valve that the surgeons refused to replace because operative failure was much more likely than success, congestive heart failure with bilateral lung and leg fluid retention, cardiac arrhythmias, and a stroke that explained the crooked mouth and the saliva that often escaped from one corner.

There he sat. Captain's hat in one hand as a reminder of past glory and a handkerchief in the other to capture the drool—a reminder to take a daily blood thinner that should guard against another stroke.

I asked, "Enough time to do what?"

"Doctor, we've known each other long enough for me to tell you that I still have fond memories of Greece. I dream of meeting younger generations of my family, returning to my village to walk its streets, enter its shops and view firsthand the transcending beauty of its nearby hills. Will you help me undertake my last great adventure—my final journey?"

I had been asked another complex question that could not be answered with a simple "yes" or "no."

"I need not remind you," I said, "that long-distance air travel is stressful. Is your return to Greece so meaningful and important in the twilight of your life that you would risk dying in the effort?"

Without hesitation, he replied, "I don't want to wait for Death to knock on my door. Let Death find me on my terms. You don't go to sea as a youth if you're timid. During my entire adult life I've been challenged by the sea. There are always risks like avoiding collisions in fog, riding out major storms in turbulent waters and encountering uncharted hazards, to name a few. Recently I've just existed in hibernation. Risk is exciting—to undertake risk is to know you're alive."

I agreed to help Panos on his mission.

Dual citizenship permitted access to Greek social and health services. These institutions helped plan an agenda. Panos was escorted to John F. Kennedy International Airport and was met at Athens. He had contact information for all doctors along his route, multiple copies of his medical records and an excess supply of medications. Monitoring of blood thinning was arranged. The duration of daily travel was restricted. Adherence to a low-salt diet was essential.

I breathed a sigh of relief when a revitalized Panos deplaned on our shores. He stopped by my office to show me a packet of soil from his village and told me that returning with the packet was worth the risk. He had plans for it that he would not share with anyone.

As predicted, within the year Death finally knocked on the door of his harbor home. Panos Panopolis was buried with the packet of village soil and his captain's hat, symbols of a proud heritage and a life lived with courage.

Jesse

His ascendance from poverty wasn't dumb luck. He succeeded because he was intelligent and was driven to make it happen. Jesse was an extraordinary man. His rise from abject poverty was based on his *Modus Operandi*—his mode of operation—which was perseverance, fairness, honesty and likability.

Jesse Collins grew up in the Deep South. He was the youngest of a large family whose limited resources were so far below the poverty line that it was a wonder that he and his siblings survived long enough to complete their state's minimal, mandatory, schooling requirement. His family lived in a tar-paper shack with a tin roof, on an isolated back corner of their one-acre plot that was laden with crops of varied vegetables for market and their own table.

Although underfed and undernourished, he and his family were seldom ill. They all had a strong constitution, high-level energy and innate intelligence. Those characteristics didn't help when lack of opportunity kept them wallowing in poverty.

Young Jesse graduated high school during the Great Depression. There were no jobs to be had in his rural town and his only marketable skill was self-taught carpentry. He imagined that there were more opportunities up north. So, at age 16, he bid his family farewell and set out in hopes of having a roof overhead and some food in his stomach.

He lived the life of a hobo—and "rode the rails" to Providence, Rhode Island, when it was enduring a brutal winter. He slept in Roger Williams Park covered by a blanket of newspapers and an outer quilt of snow. Finding a job, any job, was essential. There was no time to waste. There was no time to beg for a cup of coffee or to ask, "Brother, can you spare a dime?"

Wherever his intuitive compass directed, Jesse asked for steady work or any type of odd job. There were few odd-job takers until he got a break while walking through a commercial district. A trailer truck pulled out of a garage, and the garage's vertical door remained open. Jesse looked into the cavernous area. Therein were stacks of boxes and a broom on the periphery of a floor loaded with litter. Seeing no one in sight, he grabbed the broom and furiously started to sweep the litter into piles, picked them up by hand and placed them into an empty trash barrel. He had almost finished the job, when he heard a voice.

"Hey, what the hell are you doing?"

"I'm cleaning up this mess."

"Who the hell are you?"

"I work here."

"Like hell, I'm the boss."

The charade was exposed. So Jesse explained his circumstances, his hope of finding employment, and if there wasn't an opportunity here, perhaps he could be paid something for his partial cleanup.

The boss listened, looked Jesse over several times, must have seen an interior goodness within the exterior grime, and extended his hand.

"I'm looking for a handyman who's a good worker. You'll do if you don't mind living in the loft over the back wall of this place." As he finished the last word, the boss turned and pointed to the spot.

That's how Jesse made his good luck happen. That's how he found employment with the Empire Fixture Company. He rose in the organization from handyman to carpenter, to designer of display cases and finally to supervisor of installations. In that capacity, Jesse was sent to plan and complete an installation for a baked-goods shop in Lenox, Massachusetts. The result so pleased the owner that he persuaded Jesse to leave Empire with an offer that couldn't be refused. The new job was to plan, design, install and maintain the needs of a chain of bakery outlets that was projected to encompass New England. Jesse's skill set enabled him to do far more than keep a roof overhead and avoid starvation. He became financially comfortable and had a happy marriage.

We met when Jesse was in his mid-sixties. His problem was an all too familiar complaint of text-book-variety exertional chest pain that is associated with coronary artery disease, commonly termed angina or angina pectoris. For many months, Jesse ignored the problem when it presented and even after it persisted for many months in a mild and infrequent form. Now, stoical Jesse sought relief because symptoms were interfering with his work.

There was adequate scientific evidence that tobacco was a killer, and Jesse's addiction was in the process of doing just that to him. My medical management was conventional. It included a cardiac stress test to confirm the diagnosis, followed by coronary angiography that demonstrated diffuse disease, followed by triple-bypass coronary surgery. All went well without complications. Return to work without chest pain was a welcomed change. Cessation of smoking was an unwelcome suggestion. In a compromise that was agreed upon between a grateful patient and me, smoking was reduced from two packs a day to one pack per day.

Arterial disease is seldom confined to a single vascular bed. Coronary arterial vascular disease is often associated with cerebral, renal or peripheral vascular disease. Not long after angina disappeared, exertional right-leg pain presented. At first the discomfort was mild with a need to slow the pace until the pain disappeared. Moderate-rate ambulation usually caused moderate "claudication" pain in the lower leg; in the calf muscle to be precise. Jesse tolerated the discomfort and its possible consequences for three years. Addiction to tobacco aggravated the problem by ensuring progression of diseased leg arteries. Eventually if Jesse walked at a moderate pace, he had to completely stop until the pain disappeared. When he stopped, awaiting pain relief, there was nothing for an addict to do other than light up another cigarette. Fortunately, pain did not occur while walking very slowly at nearly a snail's pace.

Eventually, right-leg pain not only limited Jesse's ability to walk more than thirty yards, it also limited his ability to work. After two failed attempts at right-leg arterial bypass surgery, Jesse was desperate. The concern, the discomfort and the tobacco had exacted their toll. He looked worn, with greying hair on a balding scalp and drooping lids that half-covered his sunken eyes.

We discussed past medical and surgical failures to relieve his claudicated leg. He could not stop smoking and did not want to quit work. He asked about other management options.

I answered, "There are two options. The most reasonable is to retire from work. The least reasonable is to have a below-the-knee amputation that might kill you."

Most choices in life are influenced by past experience, so Jesse Collins' prior journey through life would determine his decision. We are a composite of our present and past circumstances.

I paused, waited several minutes, then asked,

"Well Jesse, what's the verdict?"

"Schedule the amputation."

"If you survive, why do you believe that you'll be able to manage the work load with an artificial leg?"

"I'll be able to work because I know someone who had the same operation, then a prosthetic leg, and still plays basketball."

"Wow that's something. How old is that person?"

"Oh, that guy is much younger than me. He's about 28 years old."

I'd hit a dead end with Jesse. He was determined to have his emotional agenda override reason, so I tried another approach.

"Jesse, have you activated your Social Security Benefits?"

"Yes, this year."

"Are you in a financial position to retire?"

He looked toward the ceiling while his brain became an adding machine, muttered some words like "no mortgage," "rental property," "retirement plan" and "bank savings." Then he looked me in the eye and said, "Yes, I am, Doctor. Try to understand. No one in my family ever retired. We work until we drop."

His next words were: "Schedule the amputation!"

CHAPTER SIX
The Tyranny of Guidelines

Introduction

Today's doctors struggle to have self-determination in managing their patients. They are restricted by guidelines that are promulgated by specialty organizations based on evidence published in the medical literature. The guidelines are extremely helpful. However a physician may be "guilty" of not following "best practices" because a patient refuses to go along with the published recommendations; or because the doctor chooses among controversial guidelines issued by opposing cross-specialty organizations; or because a wise physician, with a long past experience of success, chooses an approach that has not been thoroughly studied. Any of those scenarios place the physician at risk for poor practice and denial of reimbursement by a health insurer.

In today's repository of Internet-based medical knowledge, a patient might have a better understanding of their problem than their primary physician.

Prostate cancer is the most frequent form of cancer in men. One in six men in the US will have a diagnosis of prostate cancer in their lifetime.[1] In 2014, 223,000 men were newly diagnosed with prostate cancer and 29,480 died of the disease.[2] Doctors have two common methods of screening for prostate cancer. One is a digital rectal examination of the prostate gland that relies on identifying a lump, bump or unusual area of hard texture, and the other is a more reliable Prostate Specific Antigen (PSA) chemical blood test.

The U.S. Preventative Services Task Force published several recommendations that have been adopted as guidelines by specialty organizations; the first in 2002, the second in 2008, and the last in 2011. It is currently gathering opinions for another publication.

The first guideline suggested that further diagnosis and treatment (biopsy, surgery, hormonal therapy or radiation) based on an elevated PSA might be harmful.[3] The last in 2011 (an extension of the 2008 recommendation based on probable but not absolute evidence) unequivocally recommended that all screening be discouraged, including healthy men age 50-69. The Task Force believes that most men with prostate cancer aged 70 or older will have a low-grade localized cancer that will remain unchanged, and the majority of those men will die from causes unrelated to their prostate cancer. The Task Force concedes that men of high risk such as African Americans and those with a strong family history could continue to have screenings.[4]

The recommendations could prevent unnecessary harm in the majority of men, but could lead to premature death in a minority.

There are some facts that primary physicians should keep in mind:
1. More than half of all cancers occur in patients 65 years or older.[5]
2. As men age, the likelihood of low-grade localized prostate cancer increases. At age 50 there is a 30 percent chance; at age 70, a 50 percent chance; and at age 100, a near 100 percent chance.[6]
3. Not all specialty organizations agree with the Task Force recommendations. The American Urological Association, the American Cancer Society and the American College of Physicians believe that a discussion should occur with each patient before a final decision is made about prostate screening.[7]
4. It is said that some doctors have become confused by changing U.S. Preventive Services recommendations.
5. On April 11, 2017, the Task Force issued preliminary draft guidelines condoning a doctor-patient discussion about screening between age 55 and 69, but stating there should not be any screening of patients who are age 70 or older. However after a 20-year decline in the incidence of prostate cancer, the rate of advanced disease has risen, possibly because of a sharp reduction of PSA screening. In May of 2018, the Task Force recommended

that all patients between ages 55 and 69 have a doctor-patient discussion about screening.[8]

Some doctors are misinformed; others mismanage their patients' fears about having prostate cancer. Some patients are told that the PSA is inaccurate or that there is no need to worry about having prostate cancer.[9]

A trio of stories about patients with concerns regarding prostate cancer, their management and their outcomes follow.

End Notes

1. Screening for Prostate Cancer: U.S. Preventive Services Task Force Recommendation Statement. Ann Intern Med 2008; 149(3): 185-191
2. Gulati R, Tsodikov A, Etzioni R et al. Expected Population Impacts of Discontinued Prostate Specific Antigen Screening. Cancer 2014; 120(22); 3519-3526
3. Harris R, Lohr KN. Screening for prostate cancer: an update of the evidence for the U.S. Preventative Services Task Force. Ann Intern Med 2002; 137(11): 917-929
4. Chou R, Crosswell JM, Dana T et al. Screening for Prostate Cancer: A review of the evidence for the U.S. Preventative Services Task Force. Ann Intern Med 2011; 155: 762-771
5. Edwards BK, Noon AM, Marriotio AM et al. Annual Report to the Nation of the Status of Cancer, 1975-2010, Featuring Prevalence of Comorbidity and Impact of Survival among Persons with Lung, Breast, or Prostate Cancer. Cancer 2014 May 1, 1014 DOI 10.1002/cacr.29509
6. Berg AO. Screening for Prostate Cancer. Letters 16 Sept, 2003. Ann Intern Med 2003(6): 532
7. Gulati R, Tsodikov A, Etzioni R et al. Expected Population Impacts of Discontinued Prostate Specific Antigen Screening. Cancer 2014; 120(22); 3519-3526
8. Prostate cancer rate stops decreasing. The Boston Globe; May 23, 2018: A2
9. Tanaja SS. Editorial comment J Urol 2016; 195(2):350-51 Re: Drazer MW, Hou D, Eggener SE. Re: National Prostate Screening Rates after the 2012 U.S. Preventative Services Task Force Recommendation Discouraging Prostate-Specific Antigen-Based Screening. J Clin Oncol 2015; 33(22): 2416-2423

Jim's Prostate Cancer

Jim was raised on a tobacco farm in the Deep South, volunteered for military service and attended optometry school. His intelligence, demeanor and work ethic landed him a job at a prestigious university eye clinic.

He tells people that I twice saved his life. The first time was when he came under my care with pulmonary edema and a rapid life-threatening heart rhythm. An implanted pacemaker-defibrillator and medications got him back to work. The second time occurred years later when I cared for him during an episode of near-fatal, bilateral, pulmonary emboli.

Jim's PSA level was mildly elevated. A urologist was consulted. Prostate biopsies revealed a low-grade cancer. Surgical removal was recommended, but Jim opted for watchful waiting. The decision had merit, for his occasional PSA blood tests remained stable for the next 12 years. During the last three of those years the prostate enlarged and partially obstructed urinary outflow from the bladder. A medication (Finasteride) was prescribed to shrink the prostate. Jim was pleased with the result.

Then, a controversial U.S. Preventive Services Task Force guideline was published. It discouraged the performance of PSA blood tests on the asymptomatic elderly. Doctors were advised to be circumspect in proposing procedures to eliminate prostatic cancer because asymptomatic patients who had procedures and treatments based on an elevated PSA often had adverse complications. Treated patients did not live longer than patients with elevated PSA levels who remained asymptomatic on a program of "benign neglect" of their unbiopsied-untreated cancers. Many doctors disagreed, but Jim's doctors followed the guideline for the asymptomatic and the elderly. There were no PSA tests for three years. The next test result had a dramatic elevation that was almost off the charts. Even though the PSA had rocketed up, Jim remained unconcerned and without symptoms. However, when the urologist found a rock-hard area on the prostate, Jim reluctantly agreed to further studies.

A bone scan revealed multiple areas of likely cancer that had spread from the prostate to the skeleton. A prostate biopsy revealed the highest grade of cancer.

A 2013 scientific study concluded that patients taking Finasteride were more likely to develop high-grade prostate cancer than those patients who were not receiving that agent.

When there is a troublesome outcome, most doctors review the patient's course and the actions of the medical establishment. In this case they might ask, "Would Jim's health-and-wellness scale still be in balance if annual PSA studies had been performed? Would the spread of cancer have been prevented with earlier diagnosis and treatment?"

When tumor-shrinking chemotherapy was proposed, Jim did not want to undertake treatment if side effects would immediately make him ill. He was content to enjoy his asymptomatic state and delay any consideration of treatment until the cancer caused pain or suffering. If such occurred, he would face that challenge and prevail. Jim was resilient, having overcome serious medical illness and personal troubles in the past without falling apart.

After I retired from clinical practice, we stayed in touch. When asked to accompany Jim to a meeting with his urologist, I agreed to do so as a friend. Time and space do not alter the strong bonds of long-term patient-doctor relationships.

The urologist's seemingly prepared talk ended with a request for Jim to start a relatively benign oral medication that should delay symptoms, should be well tolerated and should have the potential to significantly shrink the tumors. During the monologue we listened and I nodded my approval when Jim agreed to be treated.

At this writing, Jim remains asymptomatic with evidence of tumor regression. We will await the outcome together.

A Patient Without an Advocate

Philip was a successful industrial engineer who had ascended to head his family's international corporation. He was groomed for leadership at a young age. Philip had all the essentials for the role. He was a superior athlete, possessed exceptional intelligence and creativity, and assumed a leadership role in any group where a collaborative effort was required to solve a problem.

He was a privileged youth from a wealthy family. His parents were mindful of not "spoiling" Philip or his younger sister Maria. They were schooled in the importance of education, virtue and to never compromise on principles.

As a youth he attended an elite private preparatory school in Connecticut, was captain of the football and baseball team in his junior and senior years, class president all four years, valedictorian at commencement and was voted "most-likely to succeed." Philip and his date were the King and Queen of the senior prom. They looked like a pairing put together by a Hollywood casting director. He was six feet tall, brown eyes, a broad smile and light brown hair. She was slightly shorter, blue eyes, dimpled cheeks and blond hair.

He went on to Massachusetts Institute of Technology (MIT) and after graduation worked at a branch of his family's industrial-engineering empire in Germany before returning to Cambridge, Massachusetts, where he was on the faculty of MIT. As an engineer, Philip was very meticulous. He approached a problem like a master chess player. Every move was well planned for safety and efficiency. That might be why—with his approach, intelligence, and creativity—he independently invented and patented a hydro-electric generator that was far more advanced than any predecessor. The generators were manufactured by his family and installed in hydroelectric dams throughout the world. Philip proudly mentioned that no other generator compared to his, and that no intelligent hydroelectric dam architect would consider any other generator than his. In that regard he told me, "I have the world by the balls."

We met when he was 66 years old. He was referred by his internist because of palpitations from a so-called atrial arrhythmia (an abnormal rhythm that originates in the small chambers of the heart). Philip's lifestyle, as an industrial leader, academician and engineering scientist was hectic. There were too many commitments each day that resulted in too little sleep, too much caffeine and too much alcohol in the course of hosting others or being a guest of honor.

Philip was overcommitted. He had little time to focus on his health. Spare time was at a premium, so for two years he had been under the care of a concierge-doctor-internist who would see or speak to him on demand.

The palpitations almost disappeared with adherence to my recommendation for changes in lifestyle. The most important were limited alcohol, regular coffee only with breakfast, and at least seven hours of sleep. However, when the disquieting palpitations returned, I was once again interrogating Philip as we sat facing each other in my office. A probing history revealed that the likely cause of palpitations was triggered by two events. The first was the painful death by prostate cancer of a long-term friend, and the second was an unpleasant anxiety-related event caused by his concierge primary-doctor's refusal to order a prostate-specific antigen screening blood test (PSA) based upon the doctor's likely misinterpretation of a governmental guideline that discouraged, but did not preclude, such screenings. Philip's view was that he was paying a premium to be included among the patients in the concierge practice, and that he felt strongly enough that he would pay out of pocket for the test if it was not covered by his medical insurance. Yet the primary doctor insisted that he was in charge, knew what was best for his patients and would not order the test.

It was my responsibility to mitigate the cause of the benign palpitations by reducing Philip's anxiety about not knowing the status of his prostate. If I did not take some action, Philip, with his intelligence and problem-solving capabilities, would eventually find a way to have the PSA test. The least I could do was to screen for prostate pathology by the time-honored method of examination of the prostate gland with a latex-glove-covered finger via a rectal examination; a procedure that had never been done by the concierge internist. The examination revealed that the prostate was asymmetric. The smaller portion was smooth and the larger portion was nodular. Based on my findings, I recommended that Philip see a urologist for further advice. The urologist repeated the examination, confirmed my findings and agreed that it likely represented prostate cancer. When the PSA result was elevated, his suspicion was confirmed. The next step was a biopsy that revealed evidence of moderate-grade cancer. After extensive imaging studies, the cancer was determined to be stage two—still localized.

A potential life-threatening diagnosis was established and a treatment plan with "radio surgery" radiation agreed upon. For Philip, and many others, knowledge is empowering. By knowing his status, anxiety and the palpitations evaporated.

Philip detached from his concierge doctor to be under the care of another.

Doctor, Treat Not Thyself

A glorious sun-drenched fall day was in view beyond the window in my office. It was Saturday morning; the patient had not yet arrived. So toward the end of an exhausting week, I peered out the window at the pedestrian and vehicular activity, preferring to be there, rather than here. A primary physician in the community had requested that I consult on a senior pathology professor from a nearby medical center. His problem was recent exertional chest pain while jogging. Symptoms were reproduced during a stress imaging study that revealed a mild regional cardiac abnormality.

Professor Dudley Warren arrived late, apologized, removed his full-length overcoat, stretched to his over six-feet full height and settled into a chair. The Saturday visit was arranged for his convenience. It was his day off. Many academicians choose to receive care from doctors that are not affiliated with their medical system. Word of illness inevitably spreads along the grapevine. Privacy is often compromised. Far less chance if care is rendered at a distance from the workplace. So it was with Dudley Warren.

From across opposite sides of the desk, we casually observed each other. Most of his ruddy, weathered face was exposed under a crown of gray hair that crept down along extensive sideburns.

I asked the professor how he wished to be addressed. "Dr. Warren, of course," he replied. His demeanor exuded an authoritative air that probably had been nurtured in youth. Long-term studies concluded that tall boys with an interchangeable first and last name are destined for success.

I further observed that there were "crow's feet" at the corners of his blood-shot eyes and that the wrinkles on his lips disappeared as he explained why he had overslept, and how he had raced across town for our appointment.

At noon the previous day, Warren learned that he was to be honored for his meritorious research at a forthcoming international pathology meeting in Paris. The announcement was a just cause to celebrate late into the night with colleagues. Many toasts and many drained glasses of champagne were well deserved after so much hard work and untold hours in the laboratory.

I interrupted Dr. Dudley Warren, "No need for an explanation, I understand." I had reviewed the medical records in advance of the visit. That helped while taking the cardiac history. Warren was 72 years old. He had been a lacrosse player as an undergraduate at Johns Hopkins University, and he currently exercised by jogging along a scenic stretch of the Charles River or by sculling on the river. There was no history of premature coronary disease, smoking or hypertension. Recent laboratory studies indicated an elevated lipid profile. Medications included multivitamins in the morning and a lipid lowering "statin" each evening.

The physical examination revealed the slow pulse of an athlete, normal blood pressure, a faint ejection murmur over the aortic valve area and diminished peripheral pulses.

Before instructing Dr. Warren to remove his examining robe and change back into his street clothes, I mentioned that a review of his record never documented his having a rectal exam to evaluate evidence of gastrointestinal bleeding, a rectal mass or prostate abnormalities. In fact, there was no record of a prostate-specific antigen (PSA) determination.

Then I suggested, "If that is the case, with your permission, I can do a rectal exam now and schedule the PSA test at your convenience."

"Correct, there is no indication of what you speak of in the record because I refused to consider them. After I change into my clothes, I will explain," he replied.

I returned to the consultation room wondering what explanation might be forthcoming. I had undergone four postgraduate years of general medicine before specializing in cardiovascular disease. If a patient's internist had not performed a simple screening test, I felt obligated to do so; for little time is required to examine the interior chambers of eyes with an ophthalmoscope, or the ears with an otoscope, or perform a breast exam or a rectal exam. Like a bad dream, I had a recurring memory of presenting a case to an instructor when I was a medical student. At the conclusion, he exclaimed, "Oh my, the poor devil has a melanoma cancer of the right eye retina!"

"I didn't say that."

"You didn't look into his eyes. How do you know that a cancer doesn't lurk there?" Lesson learned, never forgotten. In medicine there are many more "sins of omission" than "sins of commission."

Once again Dr. Warren and I were seated across from each other. He addressed me in his authoritative voice. "Off the record, my chart is intentionally incomplete. Two years ago, I presented a paper at a pathology meeting in France. While there, I experienced rectal bleeding. My friends insisted that I be examined by a gastroenterologist. One thing led to another. A colonoscopy was performed and a bleeding cancerous large polyp was removed. I did not want the problem to mar my record of good health because I was being evaluated for a large life-insurance policy. I personally paid for the care received in France and "Deep Sixed" the incriminating evidence. I am about to schedule a followup medical visit in France, but will coordinate that with my impending honor."

I asked, "Did they check your prostate at the time?"

His eyes narrowed, "Gastroenterologists never do that, and don't you consider doing so because I will refuse."

Dr. Warren expounded on his point by telling me that he had performed countless autopsies on elderly men and had often found localized low-grade prostatic cancer that would most likely remain unchanged for decades. He ended with, "I know that it would be pointless to screen me. Anyhow, at my age screening is out of the question."

I retreated to my primary role as a cardiologist and told Dr. Warren that his angina chest pressure was caused by mild, non-threatening coronary pathology. The murmur over the aortic valve area and the diminished foot pulses were of no immediate concern.

I advised Dr. Warren to take a higher statin dose, to take a low-dose aspirin every other day and to carry sublingual nitroglycerine just in case unprovoked or unremitting angina occurred. Finally, exercise should be continued within the limits of comfort. As was my custom with a patient who had never taken sub-lingual nitroglycerine, I then had Dr. Warren return to the examining room and lay supine on the exam table. A nitroglycerine tablet was placed under the tongue; the blood pressure was then checked lying, sitting and standing. It was adequate and fairly steady while standing. No danger of an excessive lowering that might provoke a fainting spell. We then returned to the consultation room.

Dr. Dudley Warren thanked me, put on his overcoat, shook my hand and departed. As I was dictating a note to the referring doctor with a copy to Dr. Warren, he reappeared, told me he forgot something. I looked about and didn't see an unfamiliar item to be reclaimed.

"I forgot to remind you that our relationship is privileged and private, as are all doctor-patient relationships. I told you that I do not want anything about the medical problem that occurred in France in your record. If it does appear, or if you ever tell anyone about it, I will sue you for breach of privacy. Do I make myself clear? Do you understand?"

Pretending to be unperturbed by the demand for censorship, I reassured Dr. Warren that his reminder was not necessary; the information was originally offered "off the record." I understood and would comply.

He returned twice more for an annual cardiovascular examination at the request of his primary physician. The only change was occasional minor palpitations provoked by alcohol. On each occasion, I dutifully inquired if there had been a change of mind about submitting to prostate screening tests. It remained out of the question. On the last visit, I was bluntly told by Dr. Warren that his views, based on personal experience, had been substantiated by a government agency's blanket recommendation that screening be abandoned in the elderly. I dutifully recorded Dr. Warren's refusals to consider prostate screening. I was not under his personal threat in doing so.

Several years after I retired, sad news was whispered throughout the covert intracity medical network that Dr. Dudley Warren had metastatic cancer and was suffering from excruciating pain. I privately wondered about the source and speculated that it might be from the bowel-cancer cover up.

Dr. Warren's obituary listed his many accolades and a sentence that prostate cancer was the cause of death. I was sad. Dr. Warren's death might have been prevented

Doctor, treat not thyself.

CHAPTER SEVEN
Directives

Introduction

Many individuals do not inform family members about their preferences if their health becomes severely compromised. It is a disturbing but essential topic to chat about. At times, circumstances require a decision to save a life, to support a life or to provide comfort to a life that is ebbing and will soon extinguish. Western Society has judged that patients should pre-determine their own fate; the patient—not the doctor, and not a family member. The medical establishment that cares for patients, exists for their patients, and it is the patients who should provide a road map for their own management. There must be a discussion between the patient and the doctor. Time must be set aside for a full discussion, or several discussions. The individual must appoint surrogates (family members or close friends) to speak on their behalf if they cannot speak or otherwise make their wishes known. There must be a discussion between the individual and their surrogate. The surrogate, often termed "health care agent," has a weighty responsibility to accurately understand the sentiments of their charge, so there must be in-depth simpatico understanding of the issues before a life hangs in the balance.

The process usually goes smoothly. However there are many exceptions. When misunderstandings, omissions, failure to implement directives and the inability of a surrogate to decide what action is appropriate, the medical caretakers are left without guidance or with regret. The sorry stories that follow are examples of directives that were not properly implemented.

Assault and Battery

If I were alive, I'd sue that first responder for assault and battery. He and his crew beat me up. When I was alive and healthy, those in my lawyers' guild called me "a tough son of a bitch," and I took it as a compliment. That's because, as an adversarial litigator, they thought that I was brilliant. I wasn't brilliant; my success was built on long preparation. I attributed my adversaries' failures to poor preparation. If my opposition team told the judge or jury a half truth, I had no mercy in exposing them while shredding and nullifying their arguments. Yes, you can say that I was tough. It was a toughness I acquired in my youth. That difficult time of my life was recorded in my medical record by my doctor. I'll let him start from the beginning and bring you up to date.
~ Gabriel Greene

Following that fanciful depiction, let me say that Gabriel Greene was raised in Roxbury, Massachusetts. His African-American parents worked at the same upscale Boston hotel; his father as a porter and his mother in the housekeeping service. Gabe's father was a former marine; six-foot-three and 210 pounds of strong will and mighty muscle. His mother lost her former job as a librarian when she objected to being bypassed for promotion by less-qualified and inexperienced subordinates. She was blacklisted as a troublemaker. After that, the best she could do was finding a job as supervisor in her hotel's housekeeping division.

Gabe had a large frame and was powerful. He resembled his father's physical appearance and possessed the placid, gentle temperament of his mother. On an average day he was sent off to the local district school early in the morning. During the school day, he was bored. The classwork and homework were not intellectually challenging. Gabe was way ahead of his classmates, but wasn't assigned any advanced work. After school, he went directly to his maternal grandmother's home and devoured books selected from the Boston Public Library by his mother. They included European and American history, the Greek classics, Shakespeare and the likes of Ibsen and Shaw. If not for love of the written word, Gabe would have been just another Boston Public School youngster who fell by the wayside because of its broken educational system in the manner described by Jonathan Kozol in his book *Death at an Early Age*.[1] Eventually, in the late evening hours, his father or mother would stop by, collect him and bring him home to a neighborhood where there was occasional crime. On weekends, Gabe was mentored by his dad in self-defense and was given an exercise routine to maintain physical fitness.

In 1974, a Federal judge ruled that Boston Public Schools were segregated. Part of the judicial decision was to bus inner-city black kids to outlying, predominantly white schools. Gabe was assigned to South Boston High School. It was an assignment that was a probable invitation to a better academic experience and a definite invitation to trouble from some of the local kids who were racist and who appeared to be supported in their distaste for the federal ruling by the superintendent of schools. In South Boston, buses were pelted with rocks while en route from Roxbury to the high school. Windows were broken. Kids were cut by flying glass. There were security officers within the school and also on the school grounds. South Boston High School resembled an armed camp.

When Gabe was verbally bullied by schoolmates, he simply smiled and ignored the abuse. He was called a sissy for not going out for football and an expletive for just being who he was. When he complained to his father, and asked for advice, he was told, "Do nothing if it's only words, but if it gets physical—knock 'em down."

Then on one fateful end of a school day, while he walked to the Roxbury home-bound school bus, three upperclassmen on the football team hurled rocks and verbal abuse at him. Gabe dodged the rocks and pressed on. Then from the periphery of his vision he saw an oncoming object that crushed his cheek bone, the lower orbit of his eye and broke his nose. Gabe looked down at the brick that settled at his feet, then looked up and quickly ascertained from its flight direction, who was responsible and ran towards him while the villain's defenders followed suite. In a rage, Gabe pushed them aside, grabbed the culprit, smashed him face down to the ground and pulled his arm behind the back until there was high resistance. After an audible pop, there was none as it ripped away from the shoulder socket. Gabe then turned this vile person face up.

His next memory was being lifted from the ground by the police, having double vision, placed in a cruiser and taken to the hospital. He eventually learned that his strong suffocating hands had to be pried off the villain's neck before they choked off total air intake. He had no recall and forever had amnesia of that time frame. Whereas Gabe was exonerated after witnesses testified about the provocation caused by the rock and brick throwing, the primary villain never returned to school.

From that day on, no one dared bully Gabe. His double vision resolved. His facial bone and nose healed. Gabe settled in at the school and experienced the joy of learning, especially after his teachers recognized that they had an outstanding student and gave him added assignments to keep him occupied.

Merit scholarships to Harvard College and Harvard Law School followed. His career trajectory continued with a job at a prestigious Boston law firm and peaked after he left to establish his own firm. Initially, Gabe and his associates took on cases that were least likely to succeed. Among those that were rejected by the established law offices, he often found a pathway to win big. His reputation attracted better cases and then the best—those that were unlikely to fail.

As a very successful litigator, and a sought-out commodity, Gabe was able to command large fees that were commensurate with his talent, knowledge and skill. He moved to a comfortable hilltop home in a posh neighborhood in Brookline, a community adjacent to Boston.

At the height of his career, Gabe's kidneys failed. We met when he was on hemodialysis. Heart failure is often a byproduct of kidney failure. The dialysis sessions were performed at my hospital. There was precious little leeway in balancing his fluid volume. Too much caused overt heart failure; too little caused his blood pressure to plummet.

It was a long struggle with poor health, and we got to know each other well during weekly dialysis sessions. He seemed to be forever on the brink of a cardiac crisis from fluid imbalance or irregularities of heart rate or erratic heart rhythm. His athletic body deteriorated, as did his mind's ability to recall precedent-setting legal opinions. Gabe spoke about his predicament. There was no hope of improvement, only maintaining a miserable status quo that would eventually deteriorate. He decided to reduce the frequency of dialysis, to augment the number of full-time health aides at home and to have comfort care rather than be resuscitated if he were about to die. Gabe's parents were deceased; he never married and he had no children, so a plan was agreed upon with a nephew who was his closest next of kin. A document was drawn up about his wishes. It was dated, signed by Gabriel Greene, witnessed by a law partner and placed in the hospital record. Whatever is in a patient's hospital record either happened or is supposed to happen. A copy was placed in a three-ring binder at his home among entries by his aides, the home-care nurse and my scribblings when I made a house call.

On a Sunday afternoon, I received a phone call from Gabe's aide whose message in New England-rooted, idiomatic jargon could not have been more direct.

"I think he's dead as a dodo bird. He's sittin' in his chair, blue, bug-eyed and not breathin'."

"Don't panic. I'll be right over to pronounce him and fill out the death certificate. Whatever you do, don't call emergency services."

"I already done it."

"Then tell them to do nothing. He's not to be revived. I'm on my way."

When I arrived, there were two emergency vehicles parked in front of the house.

The aide, her ample body covered by a white apron, was waiting for me at the front door.

"I blocked the door. They wouldn't abide by me. They brushed me aside and rushed in."

The scene was terrible. Gabe was on the floor. His clothes cut off except for his boxer shorts. A burly perspiring man on his knees was pushing on Gabe's emaciated chest, an endotracheal breathing tube projecting from his mouth being tended to by a technician squatting by his head. Another sweat-drenched technician was trying to run an intravenous tube through the collapsed dialysis shunt in his arm and there was the odor of burnt flesh from unsuccessful attempts to electrically shock-terminate ventricular fibrillation—the cardiac arrhythmia that ended the life of Gabriel Greene.

I processed that scene in a flash and to no avail shouted, "Stop. Halt." Then I loudly asked, "Who's in charge?"

Someone pointed to a man in a neatly pressed black uniform standing at the periphery who appeared to be calmly supervising the frantic activity at his feet. I rushed over to this grey-haired guy with Hollywood-style rose-colored glasses.

"Stop! This man isn't to be resuscitated."

The supervisor momentarily glanced at me and then turned back to the gruesome proceedings.

"Who are you?"

"His doctor."

"How do I know? Let me see your credentials."

So I pulled out my wallet and waved my medical license and my hospital employee card under his nose.

"Well I'm in charge, not you. How do I know he's not to be resuscitated?"

"Because I say so and there's a certified order by his bedside."

"Show me."

"That deaf haddock wouldn't listen; I told him about the certificate when he barged in," interjected the aide.

So, I rushed to the bedroom, picked up the binder and showed the document to the supervisor. He looked from the document to his hyperactive men.

"Are you guys making any progress?"

"No. No signs of life."

"Then call it off."

The Hollywood stand-in held my elbow and escorted me to an empty room.

He took off his glasses, looked at me with downcast eyes and quietly said, "Sorry, Doc, we're just doing our job. We've been sued twice for not resuscitating a person after listening to a family member or someone who claimed to be a doctor. We have to find a fail-safe way to protect our organization and your patients."[2,3]

End Notes

1. Kozol, Jonathan. Death at an Early Age 1967, New York. Plum of the Penguin Group.
2. Lown, Bernard, MD. The Lost Art of Healing 1996, Boston. Houghton Mifflin Company; 280-282. A similar unwanted resuscitation of his elderly mother is described by Bernard Lown, MD. His efforts (and mine) to have the emergency personnel cease their revival efforts, were ignored and futile. His mother's location is not mentioned, but the town might have been the same.
3. Gabriel Greene died at the age of 45 in 2005. The next year the Massachusetts Legislature passed a DNR (Do Not Resuscitate) Identification Registration Law that should protect patients, who wear a unique wrist band, from being resuscitated by first responders.

When Good News is Bad News

For three days he was a fixture in the waiting room adjacent to the Medical Intensive Care Unit (MICU). He would frequently be at the bedside of his disoriented, confused and laboriously breathing mother. He would quietly speak to her while holding her hand. At other times he would go to the cafeteria for some nourishment, or visit the rest room to wash his face.

Barney Marshall's vigil had taken its toll. He looked like Hell. He had facial stubble, unkempt hair and wrinkled cloths from sleeping in a chair, or preferably on the brown leather couch when most visitors had departed.

Barney could have heeded the MICU staff's advice to get a few winks of sleep in the comfort of his nearby home. No, he wouldn't do that, knowing that death was imminent. At home, he'd just lay in bed awaiting the telephone's ring. Better to be here to kiss her forehead and hold her hand one last time while her warmth had not yet turned frigid.

His eighty-nine year old mother, Andrea, had life-long asthma with progressive pulmonary deterioration. She married late in life and almost died while delivering Barney. His father, Sebastian, was an only child. He died young from a heart attack when Barney was a teenager. For years, Barney had nightmares that he was destined for an early death; he would follow in his father's footsteps. "Like father, like son." Barney was a nervous, distracted youth. His widowed mother had been delivered a broadside when Sebastian died. Ill prepared to support herself; she barely survived on Social Security entitlements after a kindly landlord lowered her apartment rental payments. Barney performed poorly at school, partially because of constant nightmares, distracting thoughts about having enough money to acquire the basic necessities of life and his mother's seemingly total reliance on him for everything—because she appeared incapable of formulating any plans for the business of life and living. In time, Barney came up with a plan of his own. He enlisted in the Army. As the only bread winner in the household, he knew that if things got worse for his mother, he could apply for a hardship-dependency discharge. Barney transferred the majority of his paycheck to his mother. Military admission tests indicated that he had an aptitude for technology. The outcome was an assignment to a technical unit where he could be trained and be in a position to be employed when his tour of duty was over. The plan worked wonders.

"Like father, like son" had a thread of predictive truth for Barney, for he too was diagnosed with coronary heart disease. That's the reason we had met, nine years previous. He was now in his mid-fifties, had modified his health habits for the better and had far less angina. I suggested that he reduce the stress of his job, but he was unable to get his boss to change his job description which was a highly paid technician, a trouble-shooter for an international company that made robotic machinery to replace manpower. Whenever a robot failed at any point on the globe, and a simple fix didn't cure the malady, Barney was ready to make a "house call." His unstable home life, living with and supporting his mother, permitted limited opportunity to fully tend to her needs. Her past behavior of leaning on Barney for most everything was finally explained by her having a medical condition termed "Social Phobia." Andrea preferred to be alone. She panicked in social situations. She only felt secure in her own home, or with familiar persons. Whenever Barney returned home from work, it was a wonderful reunion between Andrea and Barney—between a lonely mother and her only child. During the all-too-frequent times that Barney was away, arrangements were made for familiar helpers to shop for essentials, to keep the apartment in order and to check on Andrea. Barney planned to take an early retirement. He desperately needed to make up for lost time.

I learned from Barney that he was determined to stay at the hospital until his mother died. I visited and consoled him. Andrea Marshall was close to death, and several times Barney had instructed the MICU staff that under these circumstances there was no need to start life-support systems. She had remained in the MICU because Barney could visit at any time; her long-term pulmonologist was administering and attending to all of the patients in the MICU that month and receiving care from people whom she might recognize would prevent her from having phobic terror.

Barney was prepared for the fateful moment. He could weather the storm of emotions. He would remain calm when the messenger of death arrived.

An unfamiliar youthful member of the night shift was the messenger who aroused Barney from his couch slumber around 10:00 P.M.

"Your mother is failing fast."

She was cooler than usual to his touch. Her breathing was erratic and froth trickled from one edge of her mouth. He broke down. He had preconditioned himself for her death, but not for her final struggle. After standing straight for a moment, Barney leaned towards her ear, and whispered, "Goodbye. I love you." Then a quick retreat back to the safety of the brown leather couch where he placed his palms over tear-filled eyes.

Shortly thereafter, the same fresh young doctor bounced into the room and announced "Good news. Your mother had a cardiac arrest. We immediately brought her back with one defibrillation shock. She's breathing on her own."

"What? What did you do?"

"We revived her with a single electrical shock—followed your instructions. No life support systems like an intubation and a ventilator."

"You mean, she died and you brought her back."

"Yes. Good news."

Barney's face flushed. His head pounded. He simultaneously experienced chest pain and trouble breathing. He opened the little bottle of nitroglycerine that was his constant companion. One tablet—no relief; another tablet and a third without improvement.

"Can I help?" asked the young doctor, not realizing that he had provoked the problem.

"Ya, I'm having a heart attack. Get help on the double."

I stabilized Barney in the Cardiac Intensive Care Unit (CICU). We were thankful that the heart attack was mild. For 48 hours mother and son were in intensive care. When I delivered the news to Barney that Andrea had a peaceful death, he was calm. A silent prayer; then he said in measured phrases, "At last. No one should have to die twice. I'm so sad. I couldn't be by her side the second time. She died alone."

We had long discussions about his intentions being misunderstood by the MICU night staff that shock-terminated Andrea's cardiac arrest.

As soon as Barney was well, he buried his mother at a private graveside funeral. He remained despondent that his work schedule had often absented him from his mother's side and had prevented him from having meaningful friendships. It was fortunate that during his travels, he had bonded with a few friends in Canada.

The last time we met, Barney had a new job in Canada that didn't require travel. He intended to become a Canadian citizen and would be in a healthcare system that doesn't apply heroic efforts to delay an irrevocable near death.

In Barney's words, the greatest personal benefit about his move to Canada would be, "I will not die alone. When I am called. I will only die once."

Going Express

Leah was a wise, widowed mother of four and a grandmother of six. Wisdom is a partnership of age and experience. It is often said that we learn far more from failed outcomes than we learn from success. Leah had born witness to medical failings and successes, but the failures were like hot irons perpetually searing her memory.

It began with the prospect of an uncomplicated birth that resulted in a newborn death. Her previously healthy husband had successful, early-stage, bowel-cancer surgery; but he later died from post-operative disseminated infection. Then there was her demented father's need for institutionalization that nearly drove the family into the "poor house."

Leah was 84 years old and in "good health for her age." Her past medical history was more a source of conversation with her contemporaries than a problem. The list of encounters with illness included well-controlled diabetes, a retinal detachment, peripheral vascular disease and a transient stroke that completely resolved. She knew that in the darkness of the long shadow of a devastating medical crisis, she might suffer total disability and dependence.

It was the wisdom of her intuition that led to her request, "Doctor, when I go, I want to go express. Do you understand?"

"I do. If it appears that you are about to die, or if you are acutely ill without prospects of a reasonable recovery, you do not want to be placed on life supports or have active care. You only want comfort measures."

She accepted my analysis, and then turned to her oldest daughter who had silently listened to our conversation.

"You heard—express. Do you understand?"

"Yes, Mom."

I recorded Leah's wishes in the medical record and advised her to tell her other children about our visit and conversation.

It was an ironic coincidence, when months later, Leah had a severe hemorrhagic stroke, was in a deep coma and was on the edge of death. She required total care. Her children gathered for a continuous bedside vigil and to support each other. The children hoped for improvement, but were unconvinced that reflex movements of an arm, leg, lip or eyelid were positive purposeful signs. With one exception, they were resigned to follow Leah's "end of life" declaration. The exception was the youngest daughter, who had traveled from afar, was almost totally detached from the family and seldom communicated with her siblings or with Leah.

When pneumonia appeared, as it often does in cases of this nature, I informed the family and added a caveat that I did not plan to administer antibiotics in accordance with Leah's wishes.

"You must treat, you can't let her die," protested the nearly estranged youngest daughter. I supported my plan by sharing a copy of my office note that was prominently placed in the record and by asking the oldest child to share Leah's intentions with the others. The result was a standoff. The malcontent accused her siblings of not loving their mother, and threatened me with a malpractice suit if I withheld antibiotics.

Leah could not speak; she and I were at the mercy of her co-opted daughters who reluctantly went along with their contrarian sister—the one who rebelled against her mother's and my authority. So, antibiotics were administered. Leah stabilized, was transferred to a nursing home, remained in a coma and continued to require total care.

When someone wants to go express, the conductor (doctor) and the crew (family) should comply, otherwise the traveler boards a very slow train to nowhere.

CHAPTER EIGHT
The Pathologist Doesn't Always Have the Last Word

Introduction

The cause of symptoms and disease is often a construct based on experience and data. In ancient times, Galen and his theories reigned supreme. Illness occurred when the humors, (phlegm, dark or light bile, and blood) were determined to be out of balance. Later developments such as the microscope led to microbiology; anatomic study led to pathophysiology; and the stethoscope's ability to differentiate normal from abnormal lung, abdominal, heart and vascular sounds was another major step in the evolution of accurate diagnosis. But a detailed post-mortem examination of an organ or of the total body has always been the last word regarding the cause of death. Current technology provides medical specialists with an ability to look deeply within the body and to even guide biopsy instruments to sample tissue therein. Examples are x-ray imaging, magnetic-resonance-imaging scans (MRI), computer-tomogram scans (CT) and ultrasound. Yet, when it comes to the cause of death, an autopsy performed by a seasoned pathologist remains the Gold Standard. Without a tissue diagnosis, at least 20 percent of pre-morbid diagnoses are inaccurate.[1]

The cases that follow are about patients whose illnesses involved a pathologist who did not necessarily have the last word.

End Note

1. Causes of Death. http:www.ncepod.org.uk/2006/results_of_study_13.htm1

Cancer, Where Art Thou?

The elderly family physician was weary of Northeastern winters. Recreational skiing and ice skating were but memories. His joints creaked. His vision was blurred. His mind was made up. He was committed to retire and resettle in Florida. I was selected to care for several of his patients. Their medical records arrived.

The record on Eric Brahms was a puzzle. At the age of 56, Eric had a portion of his large bowel removed because of cancer. The pathology report stated that the type of cancer was adenocarcinoma without penetration through the bowel wall, but the cancer extended to both edges of the removed bowel segment—conclusive damming evidence that the tumor had not been completely removed. The medical entries, in chronological order after surgery, noted that the post-operative period was prolonged. Full recovery took months. The patient swore he would rather die than have another major operation of any kind; and in the natural course of events, without another operation, Mr. Brahms' cancer would recur.

I read on. Within six months after the cancer operation, this unfortunate man's vigor and vitality yielded to depression, cardiac disease and osteoarthritis. Intermittent office examinations failed to reveal any evidence of recurrent cancer and there was no attempt to verify the status of the remaining, potentially life-threatening problem. To compound the unusual circumstances, Mr. Brahms was unaware of his apparent good fortune. He was never told of his true diagnosis, only that he had "inflammation" of the bowel. With the exception of one son-in law, neither Mr. Brahms nor his family was ever informed of the cancer diagnosis. Shielding patients from a potentially life-ending diagnosis was a common practice at the time. Today the pendulum has swung from protecting a patient by concealing a possible fatal diagnosis to full disclosure of the facts, the options and the hard choices.

Before my first appointment with Eric Brahms, I met with our pathologist who specialized in bowel cancer. We reviewed the original tumor slides and the resected edges of the large bowel. The evidence was unmistakable. The adenocarcinoma had not been completely removed. The retained portion should proliferate by unregulated growth and cause havoc. That's what cancers do.

When I met Mr. Brahms, he was cheerful and appeared younger than his 76 years. His mind was quick and his gait slow. Before me was an ordinary appearing man with an extraordinary twenty-year resistance to the progression of cancer. On examination there wasn't a trace of cancer. Indeed, he hadn't a clue about a history of cancer and there was no reason for me to be an informer.

During the next fourteen years we developed a fine relationship. I also developed a close professional relationship with his knowledgeable son-in-law.

Eric Brahms died from cardiac causes at age 90. Did the cancer remain dormant or did it disappear? Was there a long reprieve or a cure? A limited or comprehensive autopsy should answer the question: Was there evidence of cancer, or absence of cancer? The family would not consent to an autopsy. So the question of the presence or absence of the cancer remains unanswered and is replaced by another question. Did the pathologist have the last word or did Eric Brahms' constitution have the last word?

Circumstantial Evidence

Guido's parents, Louis and Maria Bonopane, immigrated to this country from their home in the shadow of Vatican City, Rome. Louis was a stone mason who acted on a premonition to leave Italy before the Second World War destroyed Europe. They came with three children. Guido, age four, was the oldest. His sisters were Rosa, age three, and Gina, age two. In time, Guido became a professional photographer, never married, and was an uncle and godfather to a half-dozen nephews and nieces.

I first met Guido when he was 67 with new onset symptoms. During our subsequent conversations, he exposed his circumstances, his concerns and his heartfelt feelings. Not very old in years, he had experienced more tragedy than most. His mother and both sisters had perished in midlife from aggressive breast cancer. Louis and Guido, father and son, had suffered along with each victim during their course of radiation or chemotherapy. Father and son suffered in anguish as their loved ones' bodies were racked with nausea, vomiting, dehydration, fainting and emaciation. They witnessed the dying suffer from loss of hope, but not loss of faith that their suffering had a purpose known only to the Almighty.

Louis wondered if the family had a cancer curse that would infect all his children and grandchildren. Guido sequentially saw each victim pray for divine assistance that was not measurable even if it was dispensed from On High. Guido maintained his faith when his mother died, doubted his faith when Rosa died and totally abandoned faith when Gina died. When the last spade-full of earth covered Gina's coffin, he became a closet atheist. Guido stopped accompanying his father to church and never told Louis why.

As a successful photographer, he was in demand at political events, life-cycle events and for photo portraits of the wealthy and powerful. The building that housed his home and business—that enclosed a studio, camera shop and photographic supplies—was located in an area that gradually became infiltrated with drug dealers. One evening, an employee entrusted with opening and closing the studio was about to close when a few, armed, drug-crazed youths demanded everything in the cash register. The employee quickly complied.

Stark evidence from the security camera was damming—they took it all, then shot the poor chap dead to avoid being identified. Then they scattered—never to be apprehended.

Four senseless deaths of God-fearing, righteous people was a huge emotional burden for Guido, as it would be for most anyone. The robbery was a call to arms. Damnation to the perpetrators, he would defend himself if they returned. So, Guido joined a gun club and became an accurate shot. After getting a gun and a permit, he no longer felt vulnerable. He was licensed to defend himself, to kill if necessary.

Often in the company of client celebrities, Guido was pictured with them on the society pages of local newspapers while at charity or fashion events. There he appeared wearing his signature black French beret, a long black cigarette holder between his thumb and index finger, a cravat about his neck and a vest with a pocket-watch at the end of a chain stretched over his portly waist. The society page was not an accurate mirror of Guido's persona. In fact he led the modest life of an unpretentious successful professional who doted on his nephews and nieces. With the security of armed protection while at work, he had few concerns until his good health started to erode with symptoms of back pain, thirst and weight loss. That's when he sought my medical opinion.

The majority of symptoms suggested late-onset diabetes mellitus, perhaps related to obesity. The physical examination nuanced that tentative conclusion, for there was a firm, left-sided, upper-abdominal mass. Blood studies confirmed diabetes, and an abdominal scan revealed a pancreatic mass. In the world of medical diagnosis, the fewer explanations for a patient's symptoms, the better. By the "rule of parsimony," a single explanation is ideal and a single presumptive diagnosis of pancreatic cancer linked Guido's symptoms, physical findings and diagnostic tests. A biopsy of the mass would clinch the diagnosis and set the stage for treatment that would have a low expectation to succeed. Any treatment option was without assurance of remission, but with assurance of unpleasant or miserable side effects that might be more severe than those of untreated cancer. In the absence of a firm diagnosis, a cancer specialist would not consider a treatment. While medical and surgical specialists discussed the possible nature of the tumor and its therapy, Guido took a position that was a stunner. He would not consider a biopsy or any form of treatment. He had witnessed too much suffering caused by useless "cancer cures" and had deeply felt the gut-wrenching result of man's inhumanity to man—a senseless murder with the unknown perpetrators still at large.

"My life is ebbing. I'd just as soon end it by my own hand in my own way, rather than have the cancer or the criminals end my life."

"What are you saying? We haven't even proven that you have cancer."

"The evidence is there, even if unproven."

"You're contemplating suicide on a hunch, not a fact. What if it's not cancer? Huh?"

Guido went silent and pointed to the door.

"You might have hopes that I don't have terminal cancer, but I'm convinced that I do. My family's cursed with cancer. So please leave me alone."

He once again pointed his long index finger towards the door.

"Whew."

The mere mention of suicide triggers a mandatory psychiatric review which Guido accepted in order to be discharged from the hospital. The psychiatrist confirmed that Guido contemplated taking his own life to avoid suffering. His method for instantaneous death would be a self-inflicted bullet to the brain. The psychiatrist concluded that Guido was perfectly rational, so he could not be involuntarily committed to a psychiatric facility. He was not a danger to others and attempted suicide, or suicide per se, was not a crime.

As Guido left the hospital, he thanked me for my years of "doctoring," and we parted. Within a week, his death notice appeared in the newspaper. I contacted his niece and learned that Guido died in the manner described to the psychiatrist. Guido had the last word, not the pathologist. Death was by suicide, not by cancer.

To this day, I agonize about the pancreatic mass. Could it have been a benign process disguised as cancer?

See No Evil, Speak No Evil, Hear No Evil

I thought the elderly woman was in complete denial when she refused to acknowledge that her right breast was distorted by an immobile solid mass. Denial is a powerful psychological defense. Invasive breast cancer affects approximately one in eight women during their lifetime and age does not confer protection.[1] I gently held the patient's left wrist and guided her pale vein-lined hand to the demarcation between soft flesh and tumor, and then over the rock-hard apex of the breast mass.

Yet, Caroline Conway insisted, "I've known my body for 86 years. There's nothing wrong with my breasts. My internist gave me a clean bill of health just four months ago and, after all, you're not an internist—you're a heart doctor in charge of my palpitations."

I soon discovered that she was an obstinate lonely widow who had outlived her only child. After her enormous loss, she picked herself up and moved on. Her resilience was driven by a strong will that was molded by her upbringing, her privileged status and an inculcated early belief that she was superior in judgment and intellect to most others. Caroline went to private preparatory schools, then to Radcliffe College where she graduated *Summa Cum Laude*.

Young Caroline was a socialite, an equestrian and intellectually curious. As a spunky octogenarian, she was convinced that cancer does not present in the elderly, and, even if such an outlandish event were to occur, she would prevail without the aid of alien medical ministrations or prayer. She would defeat the evil invader by sheer will power. It was best to ignore the existence of evil; to neither speak about it nor hear about it.

Caroline refused to have a mammogram. She did not need one to prove that the images would be normal, and if a technical error demonstrated a false abnormality, she swore that she would never agree to any medical treatment.

I could not shake her belief in the myth that breast cancer doesn't occur in the elderly, nor could her primary-care physician. So I resumed my role of monitoring the status of Caroline Conway's cardiac arrhythmias every six months and cautioning her to limit caffeinated and alcoholic beverages. She reluctantly took my advice, because when she over-indulged, her heart immediately raced for several hours.

She joked, "I should have been studied by Pavlov, my reward is to be temperate." She added, "Doctor, it is not always easy to decline a second glass of wine that perfectly complements a delicious meal prepared by an outstanding chef."

I was placed in the uncomfortable, first-of-a-kind position of having to observe the natural progression of untreated breast cancer. The tumor grew in size. The breast enlarged. The skin on the surface thickened or retracted. At eighteen months the skin was dimpled like that of an orange—like the classic description by the French *peau d'orange*. Finally, the overlying skin became inflamed and ulcerated.

During the interval between my initial discovery of the cancer and its ugly progression, Caroline was sublimely indifferent to the obvious changes. I was powerless to intervene. When a treatment was proposed by her primary physician, Caroline became angry and refused to discuss the matter. The progression was unequivocally that of cancer, so much so that when the case was presented at a combined conference of specialists, the oncologists made an exception to their firm policy by offering treatment without a tissue diagnosis.

The primary internist was at her wits' end. An offer to have a psychologic review was rejected by Caroline.

"I am not depressed, suicidal or crazy. What possessed you to have such a weird thought?"

Caroline Conway lived alone and had no family, but she had a responsive support system that would act accordingly if a compromising event occurred. She lived in an elegant hotel that boasted of several outstanding restaurants—each with room-service delivery; there was also a beautiful courtyard, a dog-walking service and pet accommodations. Being on good terms with each staff member at the concierge desk, her whims or wishes were promptly accommodated.

I seized the opportunity to pierce her defense of denial when she complained of sudden severe back pain that I sensed was a pathological vertebral fracture caused by a focus of cancer that had migrated from her breast to her spine. Caroline agreed to take one tablet a day to relieve the pain.

"Off course I will, if my primary doctor agrees."

At my suggestion, and with slight deception, Tamoxifen was prescribed. It is an anti-breast cancer medication with infrequent side effects. It worked. The pain disappeared and the breast cancer started to regress.

Caroline Conway was correct in believing that she would not die from an imaginary problem, nor did she need a mammogram or a biopsy to confirm that she was healthy.

Her cancer was not bothersome, other than that brief episode of back pain which was attributed to arthritis. Death was from an unnatural cause. On a clear sunny summer day, she tripped on a loose brick in her hotel's courtyard while rushing to keep her luncheon reservation at its Terrace Restaurant. Death occurred within minutes from a massive brain hemorrhage when her skull fractured on contact with the brick walk.

Absolute denial is an absolutely powerful defense. Caroline was spared anxiety, stress, worry, sleeplessness and distraction. She did not alter her carefree active lifestyle because she did not permit herself to see or hear of evil and insisted that her doctors not speak of evil.

End Note

1. U.S. Breast Cancer Statistics. http://www.breastcancer.org/symptoms/understand_bc/statistics

CHAPTER NINE
Suicide

Introduction

Many people living in the United States are currently deliberating whether to permit terminally-ill patients access to physician assistance in terminating their lives. Seven states have passed legislation permitting physician assistance, and other states are putting the issue to a binding referendum vote or are having the proposal debated in their legislative body. Words are important, have context and have influence. Proponents generally use the term Death with Dignity, Medication-Assisted Death or Compassionate Choice. Opponents of the measure use the term Physician Assisted Suicide. In general, candidates who qualify for physician assistance in dying must fulfill several conditions: They must have a fatal illness with no more than a six-month prognosis, be of sound mind, be consistent in desiring physician assistance to die, not have remediable depression and have a compassionate physician willing to prescribe a lethal combination of drugs to be taken by the patient at a time of their own choosing. I imagine that the final act occurs when the prospect, or the actuality, of the pursuit of life and living becomes so intolerably painful, that self-inflicted death is an escape from a personal hell. A physician cannot be present or directly involved in the final act, for euthanasia is a crime. Physician assistance in the manner mentioned is not a crime within the jurisdiction of states that have legalized the process.

Opponents of Compassionate Choice usually invoke the principal that life is sacred and its termination is the decision of the Lord. No one should "play God." Opponents of Compassionate Choice also believe that a universal morality demands abstaining from assisting a person intent on suicide. Rather, the terminally ill should be managed both medically and spiritually in their last days. The physical and emotional pain of the dying can be managed through palliation or hospice care or by formal programs that mesh both concepts. Every clinician will care for numerous patients who must make end-of-life decisions. It is a universal problem among our aging population. That's why there are a number of such stories in this book.

For millennia, most all suicides have been a private matter, unwitnessed and without assistance from anyone. In recent times, those who wish to control their departure from this life often read books published by lay organizations on how to achieve a painless death. Suicide rates increase with age, and the elderly have the highest rate.[1,2]

Narcotics for pain relief require a fine balance between comfort and conscious alertness. I continue to be troubled by a recurring memory of an event during my early training. A case of malignancy-riddled bones belonged to a patient who was my high-school classmate. During my week of hospital night duty, the usually quiet hours were frequently shattered by my classmate, waking from a narcotized sleep, screaming in pain and pleading, "Let me die. Help me die." The compassionate attending doctor had no choice but to administer incremental higher doses of intravenous narcotics. Ultimately, there was a narcotic overdose. Breathing ceased. By pre-arrangement, there was no resuscitation. Whenever I recall the sad moments of that interminably long week of night duty, in my mind's eye there is an image of a painting titled, "The Scream," by Edvard Munch, and whenever I come upon a version of that famous painting, my ears are deafened by my classmate's screams.

My encounters with three suicidal patients follow.

End Notes

1. Suicide in the Elderly. https://aamft.org/imis15/AAMFT/Content/Consumer_Updates/Suicide_in_the Elderly.aspx
2. Suicide Rates Are High Among the Elderly. https://newoldage.blogs.nytimes.com/2013/08/07/high-suicide-rates-among-the-elderly/

Attempted Suicide — Ad Seriatim

Mazy Norton, at 71, was set in her ways. Unfortunately, her confrontational, argumentative air of superiority repelled anyone with good intentions towards her. A simple conventional amenity such as, "Good morning" was countered with, "What's good about it?"

This "expert on everything" appeared to be an over-achieving narcissist intellect, when in truth she graduated with the lowest overall grade average of her high-school class. Yet, then and now, she tried to intimidate everyone with her pretense of possessing absolute authoritative information. Anyone who ventured an opinion on any subject was told by Mazy that they were uninformed, ignorant and a fool.

This blunderbuss sought me out on the advice of her astrologist. Mazy wanted to confirm that her stars were aligned properly for longevity. Long life was desirable. She sought reassurance after being told by her internist that she had two deformed heart valves that produced odd sounds. I soon learned that Mazy was a bundle of contradictions. Her wish for longevity was absurd when contrasted to eight serious suicide attempts in the past ten years. Her pretense at being brilliant was exposed by her inability to answer basic questions on some common subjects. Her insistence on being independent and living alone was incompatible with her habit of eating lunch and dinner every day at local fast-food emporiums; that her apartment was a mess and might be condemned if inspected by an agent from the Board of Health; and that she was unable to comprehend the long-term consequence of her actions.

I often questioned what early environmental forces governed her behavior. She was of Welch and British ancestry. Her parents managed a dress shop for women and were among the 500 patrons who died in Boston's 1942 Coconut Grove nightclub fire. Mazy had a brother, Rick, 10 years her junior, who was solid, was a partner in a movie theatre, was married and had two adult children. Mazy had been supported by her parents and lived with them long after she should have been on her own. Upon their death, Mazy became the sole occupant of their apartment.

Doctor, Stay By Me 131

The medical record yielded no clue why, starting at age 60, she had multiple suicide attempts. She was under intermittent psychiatric care; the records were privileged, unavailable and confidential.

Survival from the suicide attempts followed a pattern. Rick would call Mazy each evening and early morning. If there was no answer, he went to the apartment and rang the bell. If there was still no response, he entered with his key. On eight occasions, she lay unconscious on the floor having overdosed on a combination of medications prescribed by the psychiatrist and internist. An ambulance was called to assist breathing, overcome dehydration and transport her to the hospital.

When I became her cardiologist, Mazy would camp out in the waiting room long before and long after her visit. While seated or standing, she would interrupt conversations between other waiting patients. She would challenge and disagree with whatever opinions they had and in the process would verbally attack them.

After a patient mentioned that Franklin Delano Roosevelt saved the nation in WWII, Mazy strode over to the seated woman, stared her down and while gesticulating, with her long gray hair swinging in the air, loudly exclaimed, "Oh, no, he was a coward. He waited too long to enter the war. He waited until the Germans had beaten the Brits to their knees. He knew the Japs were going to attack our fleet at Pearl Harbor and he let it happen. Thousands of our people were killed. He was a bad president!"

She created so much turmoil in the waiting room, that I was forced to see her off hours.

Her heart valves were of concern. The aortic valve is situated between the dominant heart chamber and the main artery that supplies the body. It had become rigid and narrowed, preventing easy outflow from the heart. To compensate, the main chamber was pumping blood under a constant strain. The mitral valve, situated between the reservoir chamber of oxygenated blood from the lungs and the main pumping chamber, had a severe leak. The damaged mitral valve could not permit its intended function to ensure one-way directional flow to the main pumping chamber. For example, the valve on an automobile tire is a one-way valve. Compressed air under pressure fills the tire. The valve prevents the release of air from the tire. So the combined problem with the inflow and outflow valves of the main heart chamber placed it under a progressive strain that predicts future failure.

While I monitored Mazy for the symptoms and physical signs of heart failure, she volunteered that she was lonely, that she had never recovered from the loss of her parents and that she was incapable of reaching out to others or permitting anyone to help out with anything but her health. So, I was not surprised when Mazy made another attempt to take her own life. The effect of pills taken with alcohol was profound. Face down in a pool of vomit, she was more dead than alive when discovered by Rick. Her hospitalization was prolonged. I objected when Mazy was scheduled for transfer to a rehabilitation facility. There had been a constant pattern of a suicide attempt, hospitalization, transfer to a rehabilitation facility, then her signing out against advice from rehabilitation to home, followed by re-admission to hospital with another near-fatal overdose. The cycle had to be interrupted. There was a meeting among all the involved doctors, nurses, social workers, discharge planners and the psychiatrists. The psychiatrists determined that Mazy had poor "executive function"—that is, she did not realize the long-term consequence of signing out of her rehabilitation facility. The solution was a court-appointed guardian to monitor Mazy's decisions about her health and to prevent obvious bad choices.

All went well until Mazy's heart started to fail. To my surprise, she agreed to consider surgical replacement of her heart valves. A senior heart surgeon reluctantly met with her, explained the procedure, the benefits and the risks, told her to think about it, gave her his professional card and told her to call his phone number if she wished to move forward. He was of a surgical ilk that believed it was a waste of time to perform coronary surgery on a continuous smoker, to replace a heart valve infected by bacteria introduced by the bad habits of an unrepentant main-line drug addict or to have a wonderful result of open-heart valve surgery come to naught because of a suicide.

Mazy told me that she shivered in the presence of the surgeon's cold detached objectivity.

"He didn't seem to care about me. I believe he regarded me unworthy of his time or effort."

So when she backed off from having the procedure, I had a flash of insight. Mazy wanted to be cared for. When she was in the depths of her misery, it would be okay if a suicide attempt was successful and it would also be okay if it failed, for she would be cared for during the entire process of recovery. She never signed out of our hospital against medical advice, only the rehabilitation facilities. That is probably because she had to go to the first one that accepted her. She seldom, if ever, was cared for by personnel who were familiar with her confrontational conversational style and could deal with it. She needed doctors and medical personnel who treat patients in the ideal manner suggested by Dr. Francis Peabody of Harvard Medical School. His words are often quoted: "The best way to take care of a patient is to care for the patient."

After she agreed to a see another cardiac surgeon, I selected a skilled junior staff member and explained the need to approach Mazy in an unhurried manner. After several prolonged visits, Mazy agreed to have surgery. Her recovery was uneventful. She was transferred to the rehabilitation center of her choosing; into the care of medical personnel who knew her and could deal with her abrasive ways. She thrived there. So much so, her court-appointed guardian convinced her to give up her apartment and transfer from the rehabilitation section to the assisted-living resident level at the multipurpose facility where she would continue to be surrounded by caring staff members.

The plan worked. When I visited Mazy, she was no longer lonely and insecure. When I asked, "Do you ever have suicidal ideas?" she replied, "Doctor, are you out of your mind? What is wrong with you? Can't you tell that I am smarter than all the other residents here and that I'm the only one who has all my marbles? Can't you tell that I am happy here?"

Change of Heart

The second heart attack totally drained Henry Anatole's vitality. He became too weak and fatigued to maintain his dental practice. Congestive heart failure was a prime concern. Henry required constant monitoring of weight, fluid intake and outflow, salt content in food, and a strict schedule for medication.

Henry had been a sick kid with sudden, very low blood pressure termed "neurogenic syncopal fainting spells" that were triggered by emotion. The attacks were controlled, but not totally eliminated, with hydration, compression stockings and quickly sitting or lying flat on the ground at the first warning of an attack. Yet occasional crisis, and a restricted life style (avoid heights if unrestrained and never swim alone), were memorable reminders that he was not normal.

I met Henry during his admission to the Coronary Care Unit, when he had his first heart attack. While lying flat on his back in his bed, his face could be easily forgotten. It had no special distinguishing features. But when he turned his head leftward toward me, his right scalp had a previously hidden, nasty, irregular vertical scar betrayed by premature thinning of what once was a robust thatch of brown hair. The scar was a reminder that his head dragged along the corner of a desk during a fainting spell at his elementary school.

Henry's heart muscle had an abundant reserve that was nourished by relatively normal arteries. The sole coronary-artery blockage was in a small vessel that resulted in minor damage. After his uneventful recovery, I became his cardiologist and his confessor. He had dark thoughts about disability and death. After the heart attack exposed his vulnerability, Henry became a disciple of the media ministries that preached or wrote about heart health. In time, with diet, exercise and medication, he felt better than ever and never became fatigued during the long hours demanded at his dental practice.

In spite of his flight to health and in spite of his affairs being in order in the event of a crisis, Henry's dark, morbid thoughts persisted.

Hippocrates reminds us that a grievous crisis can destroy good health in an instant, and so it was with Henry Anatole. He had another heart attack two years to the day after the first. It's often difficult to know what was the precipitant of a heart attack that occurs while sleeping—perhaps a bad dream? But there was no doubt that a heart attack caused Henry's severe chest pain upon awaking. First responders arrived within minutes. The pain was so intense that Henry preferred to die, rather than endure continued agony. He passed out while trying to grab a knife from the boot of an ambulance attendant, hoping to drive it through his own sick heart. Henry woke intubated in the Intensive Care Unit. The breathing tube separating the vocal cords prevented speech. So Delores, Henry's wife and health care agent, spoke for him.

"Do everything you can. I don't want to lose him. He recovered from the last attack. He's a fighter. He'll recover again."

After that pronouncement, Dolores rolled her large blue eyes, and then closed them as if in prayer. She was petite. To compensate, her brown hair was drawn up in a cone with intent to add six inches of height.

Dolores and Henry met when he joined a three-man dental practice. Dolores was the receptionist and office manager. Their professional relationship became personal. They had been married for twenty years. There were no children.

Henry did survive, but with a severely damaged heart that classified him as a "cardiac cripple." Physical limitations were intolerable. Mental equanimity was impossible. He was brutal towards Dolores.

"She should have detached me from the ventilator," he said. "I would have welcomed the Angel of Death."

Too late. Henry was dependent on Dolores for all but his minor needs. He was confined to the upper level of their home which was located near my office, a circumstance that easily permitted me to make home visits. Henry shared his thoughts with me, but not with Delores or the visiting nurse. He spoke of being lonely, of having minuscule hopes of recovery dashed.

He frequently asked, "Why me" and "How come?"—or "Why didn't Delores follow my instructions? I would be better dead than like this."

He confided that it was terrible to be told by his internist that, "There's no realistic hope for improvement." Then Henry added, "I believe him because I stopped praying long ago."

On future visits, Henry's litany of complaints abruptly stopped. Outwardly, he appeared to be sad. Inwardly, he seemed to be troubled.

So I asked, "What's happened? You don't complain much anymore. Are you more accepting of your limitations?"

"I've got a plan that I'll share with you if you don't tell anyone."

"Okay."

"I've hidden a stash of sedatives, pain pills and other meds that I got from the office. Dolores still works there two afternoons a week. On one of those days, I'll overdose. It will appear as if I died from constant heart strain."

"I swear to keep your secret, but did you mention this to anyone else?"

"Not really, Doctor, but I've seen a psychiatric social worker who doesn't believe that I'm depressed. She knows my childhood history of unpredictable fainting, my never wanting to be dependent and my current misery."

"Contact her and tell her about your plan. An overdose might not be the best idea."

There was no response. Henry just turned toward the window.

Two weeks later, the Emergency Department paged me. An ambulance had delivered Henry in an unresponsive state. Delores was hysterical. I was needed there.

While vital functions were being stabilized with life supports, Dolores spilled out her story in spurts as she rapidly spoke and only stopped to catch her breath.

When she returned from work earlier than usual, Henry screamed out, "I'm going to die, call 911, tell them it's an emergency."

She did, and then rushed to his bedside where he confessed, "After I took an overdose, I changed my mind. Have them hurry."

Then he passed out.

When Henry recovered, he was contrite. He kept referring to himself as being stupid. He changed his mind when he turned his inward emotions outward toward Dolores.

"I'm all that she has. She's got no family. Why should I add to her worries by her thinking she's to blame for my suicide? She always does what she thinks is right."

I continue to dwell on Henry, Dolores and the web called the Human Condition that binds us together. It must be terrible to be told that there's no hope while near the tipping point on the grave's edge.

To Err is Human

The superintendent rang the doorbell again and again. He banged the knocker again and again.

"Why doesn't he answer?" asked the well-dressed insurance adjuster at the super's side. The irritated red-faced man with the deep voice added, "Maybe he forgot our appointment this morning. We made it for his convenience. Maybe he isn't home."

"We have to document the damages from the burst water pipe," shouted the super at the door, as if someone were listening on the other side. "If you don't open up, we're coming in."

With that, he reached into his overalls pocket, took out a key chain, selected the pass key and entered Dr. Hall's penthouse.

They explored the place in search of the doctor. They found him in the study, seated upright on his desk chair, head back and eyes staring at the ceiling skylight. He was unarousable, cold, pale and barely breathing.

"Poor guy, he's sick. Let's lay him on the floor and call 911 emergency services," whispered the now wide-eyed insurance adjuster.

While waiting for the ambulance, the burly superintendent noticed scattered empty prescription bottles on the desk, some labeled secobarbital and others labeled phenobarbital. Beneath them was a sheet of yellow, lined paper with writing on it. The super picked up the note.

"What does it say? Read it aloud."

"It's dated today, February 15, 1964. It says, 'To my friends and detractors. Let me explain why I have taken my own life…'"

"Hell, it's a suicide!" interrupted the adjuster. "Put the note back, don't touch anything."

He no sooner finished when the Emergency Medical Technicians burst into the room.

I learned about this chance discovery of a dying man from events written in the medical record by the first responders and emergency-medicine hospital staff. I was on duty that weekend and was called to the Intensive Care Unit to manage Dr. Hall's unexplained cardiac arrhythmias. The customary treatment of barbiturate overdose is straightforward. Support the vital functions. Breathing rate and pulmonary gas exchange were being managed with a mechanical ventilator; the blood pressure with intravenous fluid volume; the body chemistry with intravenous supplements of sodium, potassium and magnesium; the blood gases and acid/base balance had been normalized. Yet abnormal slow and rapid heart rates persisted. My patient was only 60 years old without any evidence of an acute coronary heart attack. Occasionally, his surgical colleagues visited. They stood by the bedside, held his hand and shook their heads in disbelief. I had briefly met Dr. Hall at hospital-based conferences. For the most part I knew of him by reputation. But I learned far more by speaking to his associates who stopped by to lend their support.

Dr. Drew Hall was a brilliant abdominal surgeon and master teacher, with a well-deserved international reputation. He was trained in England, came to the US for specialty training and remained. A list of his patients could fill a register of socialites, royalty, the political elite, the ultra-rich and the famous. He was a loner, without any relatives in this country. He lived in the penthouse of a prestigious building that was only a short walk from the hospital. Dr. Hall was admired by his surgical colleagues for his skills, but was also disliked for expecting all others to match his impossible standards. He demanded perfection of himself and everyone else. It is said that a genius like Dr. Hall emerges every century. He was critical of any medical error made by anyone of any station at any time in any place. He was totally unsympathetic of the sentiment written by Alexander Pope "To err is human, to forgive divine."

When Dr. Hall was not preparing for surgery in impeccable detail, or was not operating on a patient, he was searching the latest literature to add to his encyclopedic memory. He knew that he had earned the accolade of being "the best" because his innate skills were gifted. His eye-hand coordination; his keen sense of which tissues lay beneath the surface, and in what anatomic plane they resided; his visual depth perception; and his brain's ability to create a three-dimensional image of a surgical field was a rarity among surgeons. The skill set was supplemented with a memory of every described anomaly of every abdominal organ presented in text books, the medical journals and his extensive experience. When Dr. Hall entered the operating theatre, he was determined to succeed, as he was with every undertaking. That is what I learned about my patient while reviewing his records in the Intensive Care Unit and from speaking to his colleagues who came to visit with hopes of an early recovery.

The normal range of heart rate is between 60 and 100 beats a minute. A survey of Dr. Hall's recorded abnormal heart rhythms revealed a multitude of rapid and slow varieties originating in the small and large chambers. There were small-chamber salvos of 150 beats per minute and unrelated large-chamber salvos of 200 per minute. There were intermittent normal and rapid small-chamber beats that failed to conduct to the large chambers.

I noticed an unusual form of atrial tachycardia with so-called two-to-one block and an even rarer form of ventricular tachycardia that was bidirectional. Each are associated with digitalis toxicity. So I examined the medication bottles that were delivered by the first responders. No bottle was labeled with any of the "digitalis" preparations. Maybe there was a clue in the chart copy of the suicide note? It read as follows:

> To my friends and detractors, let me explain why I have taken my own life in an honorable, rather than cowardly, action. Fifteen years ago, I vowed to end my life if I was responsible for a surgical misstep that caused a compensable injury or a death.
>
> For decades I undertook the most complex intra-abdominal surgeries when and where others feared to tread—and always succeeded in prolonging or saving lives. Every operation was ultra-exciting because I knew that both the patient's and my life hung in the balance. What greater incentive for a surgeon to succeed? What greater advocate could a patient have?

During a recent surgery, I had a visual migraine event; I misidentified and destroyed a vital structure that caused a good man to suffer and die. His family suffered, will continue to suffer, and will forever mourn their loss.

My conscience judges that I am guilty of unintentional murder. I am no longer a savior. I am a shattered man whose confidence has evaporated. I cannot function as a timid, hesitant defensive operator. It is best to leave a legacy of high achievement. During tonight's last supper, my delicious desert will be with herbs and barbiturates to assure a peaceful and painless everlasting sleep.

Drew Hall, M.D. FRCS

Ha. There was no mention of digitalis, or was there?

Digitalis purpurea is a member of the foxglove plant. Any plant that is used for medicinal purposes is considered an herb. Unfortunately, in 1964, there was no antidote for massive digitalis poisoning.

The episodes of ventricular tachycardia became more prolonged and were harbingers of an episode of ventricular fibrillation, a form of cardiac arrest that ended Dr. Hall's life.

All cases of unnatural death are reported to the medical examiner who took jurisdiction and ordered a search of the deceased's apartment. Two empty bottles of "Digitalis Folia," wrapped in aluminum foil, were found in the wastebasket under the study desk.

Dr. Hall did not seek forgiveness nor did he err. When he undertook a task, he did so with meticulous preparation to ensure success.

CHAPTER TEN
Futility

Introduction

The concept of futility in the context of an ill-patient's care is a prediction that advanced medical management will not alter the outcome; that the patient will not improve or will not survive; and that life-support systems should not be placed or should be withdrawn if they are already in place. I neither believed in, nor was I guided by, the uncertain concept of futility.

The trio of stories that follow should illustrate why futility can be erroneous when applied to the care of an individual patient. Doctors should advocate for every patient, especially when there is doubt about the outcome. In a broad sense, the concept of futility is a numbers game—an average of many patients with a diagnosis and a shared set of circumstances. Each patient that a doctor cares for is a unique person with a unique outlook and with unique qualities—rather than just a number.

An Unexpected Request

The stroke was devastating. Independence was lost in an instant. An artery occluded in the dominant hemisphere of the brain. The result was paralysis of the right arm and leg, garbled speech and inability of the brain to accurately process or transmit information. If that wasn't enough, there were other problems such as inability to swallow along with incontinence of urinary bladder and bowel; the left body unable to appreciate the presence of the other half; and limited vision. This successful businessman, a leader in his field, a gifted public speaker, and sought-after toastmaster, was now beyond recognition.

The neurologists were hopeful that Duncan Rivers would survive, that the dead and dying portions of his brain would not bleed—that the unaffected portions of the brain would assume some of the functions of the lost portions, and that Duncan would eventually rise above the living wreck that was his current status. But he would always be disabled and should never be near normal.

Duncan was spared a late brain bleed that would likely have killed him. Total care was required. Physical therapy commenced. Partial return of right leg motion was encouraging.

Problems are inevitable in a person with a predisposition to vascular aging; a person who tempts fate by ignoring medical recommendations, and who fans the flames of destruction by embracing a lifestyle that adds risk. Duncan had high blood pressure, high cholesterol, a family history of premature coronary heart disease and was unable to stop smoking cigarettes. He was unfaithful to his medications. He relished salty food and often drank margaritas from a glass with a heavily salted rim.

I followed this potential medical time bomb at the request of his family physician. I counseled him on healthy heart habits. Enrollment in a behavioral-modification program was useless. Duncan's addiction to food, tobacco and gambling could not be altered. Yet the years passed without a major problem until his wife Bobbie found him paralyzed.

For many years Bobbie—a smart, platinum-blond, former fashion model—was devoted and accepting of her husband's bad behavior because, as she put it, "It made him happy."

The family had adequate financial and human resources. In addition to Bobbie, there were three grown children who lived nearby.

After several weeks, our acute-care hospital had completed its mission of stabilizing Duncan. The next step was to have him transferred to a rehabilitation facility. The family resisted. Bobbie demanded "either continued care at the hospital, or care at home." She was told by the social worker and neurologist that his care would be unmanageable at home. To attempt to do so would be futile. She would likely have to return his care to the hospital after a few days at home. Against advice, Bobbie took Duncan home. She and her family were put in touch with visiting nurses, home-health aides and occupational and physical therapists.

In the approximate half-year that followed, I often wondered about Duncan's status. Then I received a phone call from him.

There was only slight difficulty in his speech. When he requested an appointment, I selected a Saturday morning when I had no patients scheduled. I told him how to instruct the ambulance attendants regarding his delivery and return.

"I don't need an ambulance."

"Then do you need a chair car?"

"No! I'll come by public transportation."

"Are you sure?"

"Yes I'm sure."

Duncan arrived on the appointed summer day at the appointed time. He walked with a slight limp. Each word of his greeting was understood. His sunburned face attested to the fact that he was not home-bound. He had lost a significant amount of weight and did not have a package of cigarettes in his shirt pocket—a good start at a lifestyle change.

After he settled in a chair, and after a long silence, I spoke.

"Duncan, how can I help you? Why are you here?"

He surprised me with, "When can I drive my car?"

"As soon as you return to your neurologist and pass a driving test."

Duncan did just that. His vision remained modestly impaired, but that was not a disqualifier.

To rely on the concept of futility is in itself futile. There are too many exceptions like Duncan Rivers.

Will to Live

The physical wreck known as Lewis Macy suffered from long-term, bivalve, rheumatic heart disease, yet he would not consider surgical repair when he was a "good" risk for success. One valve was narrowed and the other was leaking. Each time I saw Lewis in the office or when he was admitted to the hospital with congestive heart failure, I made a point to ask, "Have you changed your mind about surgery?"

He had a scripted answer, "I won't sacrifice one day or one hour of my natural life by having a premature death during surgery."

And so it was with Lewis Macy. For several years, he was able to maintain extreme adherence to his medical regimen. He measured every drop of fluid intake and urine output. Table salt and salty food were taboo. His weight was recorded each morning before breakfast. After he could not exercise and dressing became an effort, Lewis remained in his pajamas with a bathrobe at hand if a guest arrived. His wife, wonderful Mary, fulfilled every medical and comfort requirement. She became his full-time caretaker. In addition to implementing his every whim, she assumed the role of his barber. Every day, she brushed shaving soap on his face and used a straight edge razor to eliminate his stubble. Each month she cut his thick, black hair. He was the master of the house. When receiving guests, Lewis sat in a high-backed recliner. His guest sat opposite in a low-backed chair. The bedroom was tidy. The commode, food tray and measuring bottles were tucked away in a closet.

The couple had a married daughter who helped out whenever she could take leave from her own family. Mary had abundant energy at the onset of her husband's decline. Now, years later, she was hampered by diminished strength and constant fatigue.

Over time, as Lewis' heart became progressively weaker, the risks of valve surgery increased. He was warned that surgery wouldn't be an option if he waited too long. If the risk became too high, the heart surgeons said that it would be futile to consider valve repair or replacement. After each discussion of heart surgery, Lewis would tell me to simply increase the dose of each helpful medication, add a new medication or alter the timetable that his pile of pills should be taken. Each discussion ended with Lewis having the last word.

"I do not want to sacrifice a day or an hour of my life—"

During a hospitalization that took a long time for Lewis to stabilize, I told him that I had no more to offer in the way of medication.

His surprise was obvious.

"No more to add, subtract or adjust?"

"That's right."

"Are you sure?"

"Yes."

"Well, if it's either that I die very soon or have surgery, I'll have surgery."

I was momentarily struck dumb, found my voice and then said, "I'll have a surgeon see you. But, Lewis, it might be too late."

The chief of cardiac surgery, who was the most experienced with heart valves, evaluated Lewis, and to my surprise, proposed a very high-risk procedure that was agreed to by all parties.

I had to leave town for a medical meeting on the day of the surgery. I was anxious about the outcome because the risk was so high that heart surgery bordered on futility. Upon my return three days later, I went directly to the cardiac surgery Intensive Care Unit with hopes of finding Lewis there. He was not on the roster.

I thought, "Oh my goodness—Lewis must be dead. He must have died during the operation or during the hours that followed."

I inquired of a junior staff surgeon which of the two possibilities had occurred.

He gave me a strange look, "Neither. Lewis Macy is recovering very well in the step-down unit."

When I entered his room, Lewis was glad to see me, but not as happy as I was to see him. He spoke first,

"I'm grateful that you recommended my surgery when you did. Perfect timing. God wasn't on vacation. He watched over me."

We Believe in Miracles

After several days of supportive care, the 77-year-old patient gradually slipped into a coma. She was unresponsive to external stimuli, unable to speak, without evidence of a purposeful response to command, and no longer able to safely take nourishment.

To the demographer, she was a 77-year-old wife and a mother of two grown daughters. To her doctors, she suffered from obesity, diabetes and aging of all her arteries. Those that nourished her brain and her kidneys were compromised. To her husband and daughters, she was a loving bulwark of strength and their pillar of support.

To the nurses, she needed constant attention and care; attention to monitor her vital signs; attention to turn her from side to side in bed on schedule to prevent breakdown of skin at pressure points; attention to change linens when she soiled the sheets; care to prevent aspiration of secretions from her mouth towards her lungs; and care to chart measurements of intravenous input and bodily fluid output. In totality, looking after Violet Forrest was an arduous task performed without complaint.

The neurologists observed gradual deterioration, in the context of coma, attributed to problems with the nerve network that connects important parts of the brain. They predicted, "The longer the coma, the less likely the prospects for recovery."

The coma deepened and there was no remediable neurological intervention. They advised, "Be patient, just wait and see."

Time passed and I raised the issue with the family about their wish to add or avoid life supports, if there were a crisis.

"Do everything you can," they replied.

After a few more days without change, I mentioned to the family that the neurologists believed that if a crisis occurred, the best that could be expected from a successful reversal would be further deterioration or a return to the current status of Violet being totally dependent on caregivers. Crisis intervention would not improve a thing. The neurologists predicted that it would be futile.

The husband—sad, often weeping, and red-eyed—spoke for the family as he put his hand on my shoulder, and softly said, "My wife's fate is in the hands of God. Do what you can. God will decide to spare her or take her. We pray. We have hope. We believe in miracles."

Then I placed my hand on his shoulder and softly said, "Let me know if your resolve falters. If that be the case, with your permission, I will place limits on implementing extraordinary measures."

Shortly thereafter Violet Forrest developed pneumonia. That called for another discussion. To treat or not to treat with antibiotics. The family opted to treat.

Thirty days later, there was a flicker of improvement. Two weeks after that, Violet Forrest was able to sit and converse with her family. Then she was able to feed herself.

Prayers were answered.

The family had their miracle.

CHAPTER ELEVEN
Holocaust

Introduction

National and international Holocaust Remembrance Days are reminders of the massive numbers of innocent people who were worked to death, starved to death or were systematically murdered in German extermination camps.

During my early years of training, and for many years thereafter, I cared for patients with Holocaust concentration-camp identification numbers tattooed on their arms. Even if a patient refused to speak about bearing witness to a Jewish genocide, to starvation, to death-dealing hard labor or to the extermination of men, women and children who were not members of the master race, who were never able or could no longer work for the Nazi cause —the tattooed numbers identified those who survived the carnage.

Many of the survivors had persistent demonic memories. They were suspicious, cautious, paranoid, and, if awakened from sleep, believed that members of the hospital staff were Gestapo with intent to cause harm. A majority of the Holocaust survivors suffered from persistent traumatic stress.

Today, there are many Holocaust deniers, many more who were not educated about the Holocaust and those who live in countries that regard the Holocaust as a myth that never happened.

The stories that follow should remind us not to forget.

To Life

When I reflect on the death of patient Lazar Reich, I believe that he could have been a disciple of Maimonides, the revered Jewish scholar and physician who believed that each life should be preserved at all costs to permit continued devotion to God. At celebratory Jewish events, a glass is raised by the toastmaster who invariably proclaims, "La Chaim—To Life."

My first contact with Lazar Reich occurred when I was called to the Intensive Care Unit to render a second (or was it a third?) opinion about his chances of having a successful surgical procedure. Lazar had the appearance of a scarecrow with stick-like limbs, a skeletonized chest with ribs that rapidly rose and fell, a mop of long gray hair and a white forehead that reflected the overhead lights—below were half-closed eyes and an unshaven face.

The medical record indicated that Lazar's rapid decline started after he entered the hospital with pneumonia. Three weeks later, while I was gazing at this dying man with his blue lips and purple finger tips, I wondered how much longer he could endure with barely enough oxygen to support his body's basic needs. Maybe he could find a way. Maybe I could learn if his tolerance had reached its limit. Rapid breaths prevented Lazar from speaking more than a word or two. In response to questions, he could appropriately utter or nod his head to indicate "Yes" or "No." I was convinced that his mind was clear.

The hospital record also revealed that Lazar was prone to lung infections, having acquired "black lung" disease from a decade of coal mining in his native Poland before WWII.

In youth, Lazar was a solid block of bone, sinew and muscle. He was known for extraordinary strength and endurance. When the Nazis invaded, he was captured and sent to Treblinka concentration camp where there were only two possibilities: either being murdered or forced into hard labor. Lazar chopped wood for the crematorium. The workers received no rewards. It was only a matter of time when they would drop from starvation or from exhaustion. When Lazar was later liberated, at another camp, he was more dead than alive.

My examination demonstrated severely compromised lungs that caused high resistance to blood passing through them. That, in turn, causes a heart condition termed "cor pulmonale." The two right-sided heart chambers that pump blood to the lungs are forced to work against excessive resistance, become overworked and fail over time. Treatment is focused on the difficult problem of improving lung function. Lazar's lungs were filled with coal dust that was a constant and persistent irritant. The present pneumonia was confined to the left lung, was nasty, had only partially responded to antibiotics and had inflamed the outer lining of the lung and inner lining of the chest. The space between them had filled with pus-fluid. The pus solidified, compressed the lung and caused adhesions that prevented the lung from fully expanding.

I was asked if Lazar would survive surgical removal of the solidified fluid and the release of adhesions. I believed that he might survive, but in the aftermath would likely need prolonged if not permanent dependence on a mechanical-life-support ventilator.

I gave my opinion to the primary doctor and was asked by him to return and explain my views to Lazar. I sat by the bedside and held his cold hand.

"Do you remember me?"

Between huffs and puffs— "Yes."

"Are you aware that we are doing all that we can for you, but you are not responding?"

Between huffs and puffs—"Yes."

"Would you consider chest surgery to try to improve your status?"

While huffing and puffing—"Yes."

"Lazar, would you have surgery even if you might die in the process or be permanently attached to a life-support breathing machine with a tube in your throat that prevents you from speaking?"

Huff and puff—"Yes. Yes."

Lazar's children arrived. He had two sons and a daughter. I asked them how they would advise their father about having surgery if the outcome were death or survival with dependence on a breathing machine that prevented speech and required nutrition by stomach-tube feedings. They spoke as one.

"It's his choice."

All decisions about their father would be determined by their father and if he could not express an opinion in the aftermath of the surgery, all life supports would remain in place even if he had a stroke or were brain dead. Lazar had spoken. He chose to live within every circumstance, even if he were among the living dead.

I repeatedly questioned Lazar over several days to be certain that he was determined to undergo surgery. He was. A thoracic surgeon agreed to remove a rib, open the left chest, remove the consolidated mass of pus and release the adhesions that were restricting the lung from expanding. Lazar survived with a heart that improved slightly and with lungs that needed the support of a mechanical ventilator to sustain life.

Lazar's status did not change for two months, during which time he remained alert and never complained; nor did his children complain. Ultimately, he acquired an infection caused by an antibiotic-resistant bacterium that invaded the blood stream. He suffered cardiovascular collapse and died.

The children did not shed any tears in my presence, nor did they express any regrets about their father's decision to undergo surgery. They spoke to me about the high points of his life, his charitable works and his devotion to his deceased wife and to his entire family.

No regrets. No remorse. No tears.

The obituary shed light on Lazar and his children's stoicism at a time that would be an overwhelming ordeal for most others. During the Holocaust, Lazar Reich was imprisoned in two death camps. The first was Treblinka. The Russian army was advancing towards Treblinka about the same time that Lazar could no longer perform hard labor. The Nazis tried to cover up their murderous war crimes, their—insanity, by burying the dead and transferring hundreds of prisoners to Auschwitz to be exterminated. When the Nazis at

Auschwitz offloaded their victims in single file, those who appeared able-bodied were directed to the right to work; the others were directed to the left to be exterminated. After alighting from the cattle car, Lazar entered the serpentine line of fellow sufferers and willed himself to appear strong. A Nazi official, devoid of humanity, unexpectedly beckoned Lazar to the right —to live another day. The liberation of Auschwitz and the war's end saved him in the nick of time. Lazar lived to be liberated because he never gave up hope. He never dwelled on death. He focused on survival and on living one day at a time. Death was not an option. Lazar's survival-decision coin had "Life" engraved on both sides. Whenever it was flipped, it always landed with the "Life" side up.

That is why Lazar chose to have surgery.

When the Heart Stops Beating

Early in my medical career, I believed that each illness was managed by a generally accepted formula. That was until I witnessed a tense philosophical conflict between a senior resident and a staff physician.

While I was on the pediatric service of a busy hospital, an infant was admitted with a seizure disorder that was quickly controlled with medication. The diagnostic studies failed to reveal the cause. One Friday evening the infant went pulseless and stopped breathing.

"Cardiac arrest!" a nurse called out; then she shouted, "Code Blue!"

By the time the full pediatric team arrived, the infant's lips and body were blue. Breast-bone chest compressions generated a feeble pulse. A cardiac-rhythm monitor revealed absence of a heartbeat (asystole). Not even an occasional beat; and the naked eye couldn't see any spontaneous breaths (apnea).

An intern muttered, "Bad news—asystole and apnea."

Without chest compressions, there was no pulse.

Medications to stimulate and accelerate heart beats were administered with temporary restoration of heart action and temporary resumption of breathing; then, reversion to asystole and apnea.

An external skin-surface pacer arrived and a train of electrical shocks were applied to the surface of the chest with intent to stimulate the heart within. The process resulted in a heart response to each shock that created a weak pulse. But alas, after a brief time the pulse extinguished.

The electrical system of the heart is controlled by the primary pacemaker with a safety net of subsidiary pacemakers. If the primary fails, the subsidiary pacemaker signals are at a slower rate and are generally sporadic and unreliable. Our infant's heart had a disease process that had sabotaged the primary pacer and all the substations. The entire electrical grid had been destroyed. The result was asystole.

The resuscitative effort was prolonged. Both native heart beat and pulse were generated artificially and were inadequate. The infant's blue eyes were dilated and unresponsive to a light beam either because the brain lacked oxygen or because of the side effects of the heart-rate accelerant medication. There was lack of spontaneous breathing.

Jack—the youthful-appearing, unshaven, chief resident—called off the resuscitation. After he documented the time when he pronounced the infant "dead," that declaration prompted the obstinate heart to start up. No doubt about it. The still attached cardiac monitor chirped in unison with each heartbeat. The infant heart would not quit its mission to supply the other vital organs—the kidneys, liver, lungs, bowel and the vulnerable brain.

Jack momentarily appeared stunned. Then with uncertainty said, "Resume the code, there might still be life."

Everyone responded, but to no avail. Once again there was total failure of the heart's electric grid. Asystole. Jack spoke softly. "Call off the code." He recorded the time of death for a second time.

Aaron, the supervising senior pediatrician suddenly appeared. He quickly strode across the ward and positioned himself next to Jack. He was dressed in a white shirt with silver cuff links, blue tie and a black suit. Aaron appeared to have come from some event.

"What's going on here? I was called about an infant's cardiac arrest. So I came directly after Sabbath services."

As Jack started to explain the sequence of events, "Chirp—Chirp—Chirp." The cardiac rhythm monitor announced that the heart had once again spontaneously self-started.

Jack asked, "What should I do?"

Aaron: "Why ask? Do everything you can."

Jack said, "But—"

Aaron interrupted, "Start the code, stop wasting time."

All hands responded.

Jack regained his voice, "But Aaron, the pulse barely circulates blood. It's inadequate. The body's been cold, blue, and clammy. It's obvious that life hasn't been sustained. If the brain isn't dead, it's been irreparably damaged."

Aaron's angry retort: "That's speculation." Then in a calmer voice, "Keep trying. Correct the body chemistry. Keep up the oxygen. Continue the resuscitation. Newborns and infants are the hope for the future, for this family, and for all of us. If the heart beats, there's hope. Do you understand?"

"Yes"

"Then I'll leave it in your hands."

Aaron left as abruptly as he had arrived.

When the heart stopped forever, the total resuscitation effort had lasted 3 hours and 15 minutes. Jack shook his head as he thanked the emotionally drained and physically exhausted nurses and staff for their pains.

"This shouldn't have been prolonged, but I can understand the reason why. Aaron is a Holocaust survivor. When he was in Dachau he saw more people die in one day than all of us will see in our lifetimes. Aaron believes that no one is in the process of dying. They only die when their heart stops beating forever. Until then, they are living."

Underground

This is a patient's story that evolved during many visits over many years. I have organized it in chronological order. Let me start at the beginning.

Paul Pochenski was a Polish émigré who found his way to the US in the aftermath of World War II. Muscular skeletal pains and an enlarged heart almost prevented him from reaching his sponsor, the Roman Catholic Archdiocese of Boston, Massachusetts. During the war, for many, lack of fuel and food resulted in death and near-death from exposure and starvation. During medical clearance examinations to enter the US, studies revealed that Paul's weak heart resulted from parasitic trichinosis during the war. Any food, cooked or uncooked, was at a premium in preventing death from starvation. Somehow, somewhere, Paul Pochenski must have eaten gruel that contained undercooked pork.

The Pochenskis were multigenerational tenant farmers on adequate acreage to raise wheat, cattle and pigs. They also maintained a slaughter house that served the general Christian community. The absentee owner of the farm was an expatriate who lived in Scotland.

At a young age, Paul became fluent in German and Russian, which were the languages of the two most powerful bordering countries to Poland. He also had a working knowledge of English when he graduated high school.

The residents of Paul's village were multi-ethnic and of several religious persuasions. The predominant religion was Roman Catholic, followed by some Protestant denominations. There was a smattering of Jews—mostly merchants and farm hands.

I first met 70-year-old Paul Pochenski in 1990 because of his failing heart. That was long after he assimilated into the local culture, settled in the Boston area, became a naturalized citizen and had a fine job with an import-export firm that specialized in European foods.

During the next ten years, whenever I asked, "How did you survive the war?"—Paul usually answered, "It's a long story; it wasn't only my survival, it was also about my immediate family's survival. I had to consider my wife, young son and my parents."

He usually became silent, appeared to be deep in thought, then added, "Let's leave the complicated details for another time."

Yet, during unanticipated moments, and in non-chronological order, Paul would part with a portion of his guarded past.

During the early 1930s, Paul recalled family discussions that reflected concern about worrisome happenings in neighboring Germany. Things like the ascendancy of the Nazi Party, eugenics intended to promote Arian superiority, euthanasia to eliminate "suffering" of those with physical and mental defects. The oppressive actions intensified. In 1933, the Nazi Party fired all Jews and other undesirables from educational, legal, and medical governmental agencies.

Several years later, Paul told me that "One evening there was a knock on our door. It was our neighbor, Stanislaw Kaminski, the broad-shouldered, powerfully-built elder from our bordering farm. We chatted. He told me that Germany had territorial ambitions, would become belligerent and would persecute non-Arian minorities."

Paul said that Stanislaw sighed, closed his eyes for a long moment, then continued, "I am a third-generation Pole. My great-great grandmother was a Polish Jew. My great-great grandfather was a Polish Catholic. She converted before their marriage. The German authorities consider their second generation children, including my grandfather, to be half Jewish. My father is considered to be one quarter Jewish, and I am considered to be one-sixteenth Jewish, as are my cousins who have been living with me since they were dismissed from their jobs in Germany. Anyone with a trace of Jewish blood is the same as a full-blooded Jew."

After talking about his ancestry, Stanislaw added, "I was born too soon. According to German authorities we are equivalent to beasts. We are criminals because my great-great grandfather fell in love with a wonderful Polish Jewess. My cousins who had a life in Germany were suddenly treated like criminals. All full-blooded and part-blooded Jews were permanently released from governmental agencies except those who were in the German armed forces in World War I. Imagine, all Jewish teachers, lawyers, engineers, doctors, nurses and scientists dismissed from important work. Two cousins from Germany have been living with me—a mechanic and an engineer. Since they arrived, we prepared for the worst. They built a shelter in case of emergency."

When Stanislaw stopped to take a deep breath, Paul interrupted, "Why are you telling me this sad story? Why did you call on me tonight?"

Stanislaw answered, "Paul, I will tell you the reason in secrecy. We are all considering leaving for England before it's too late. While we are gone you and your family can manage our land and farm, have access to our cattle, horses, chickens, and timber. You will receive a handsome financial consideration for your efforts. Our field hands and household help are loyal to us and will be loyal to you."

Stanislaw paused; he raised his right hand and brushed some perspiration from his forehead, then the tone of his voice became less factual and was almost pleading, as were his eyes.

"Think about my proposal," Stanislaw said, "I will show you about tomorrow. Keep my confidence. I make you this offer because I know I can trust you. You are an honest man."

Then he abruptly departed into the night.

Paul immediately discussed the proposal with his wife and parents. For Stanislaw Kaminski, desperate times were calling for desperate measures. The Kaminskis had extensive land holdings that encompassed pastures, hills, valleys, tree plots and a rim that bordered on a federal forest. The families were good neighbors. The children attended the same school and were fast friends. Each family had helped the other during crises. When Paul's young son became disoriented and lost, it was Stanislaw's hound that tracked and found the lad. When Stanislaw lost control of his tractor, overturning as it went off the road, it was Paul who extracted and brought a dazed Stanislaw to the local hospital. The Pochenskis would help their good neighbor without reservation.

The next day's inspection was unremarkable. There was a large hen house, a stable with four work horses, steers, cows and a large pigsty. The wood plots and forest had an abundant variety of trees for selective timber, and there was a recently constructed emergency shelter that was designed and built by Stanislaw's cousins, an engineer and an industrial mechanic who were evicted from their jobs in Germany.

After the Kaminskis left for England, the Polish government prepared for the worst. Conscription of healthy men into the military depleted Paul's work crew. Hearty women were willing and effective in filling the void. The government contracted for more produce from the combined farms managed by Paul who was exempt from military service after being classified as an essential produce provider. Poland was ill prepared for Germany's invasion from the west in 1939, followed seven days later by Russia's invasion from the east.[1] The Germans characterized Polish people as sub-human. Thousands died in battle or were murdered. Tears appeared in Paul's eyes when he told me, "The Germans and Russians slaughtered our men, women, and children as I might slaughter a calf."

A German military commander took over the Kaminski mansion for his headquarters and billeted his men in tents on the property. He requisitioned most of their horses, feasted on their larder and drank himself to sleep each night on their wine.

"If I supplied the commandant with delicacies, and helped to feed his officers, he did not threaten me."

The Germans had a problem governing the area. The Polish Government never surrendered. They moved into exile and maintained links to an active undercover partisan army of men and women. Most every Pole resisted in one form or another. Anyone who openly spoke Polish was a criminal subject to imprisonment or death. Poles were given no respect; after all, they were sub-human. Jews were hunted, summarily killed or sent to ghettos. Many went into hiding or joined the partisan armies that moved about in the forests. Some Jews were protected and hidden by Christian neighbors.

"Secrecy was essential," Paul told me. "I had extraordinary demands placed upon me, and extraordinary responsibility—all with extraordinary danger. The German authorities imposed meager food rations on our people. The partisans were starving in the forest. Their emissaries were in contact with me. If it were known that a package fell from my wagon at a prearranged location and was recovered by a partisan, I would dangle by a rope about my broken neck in the public square."

Paul paused, and for reassurance stroked his neck before continuing. His next words were spoken very slowly to emphasize their importance.

"There were informers everywhere looking for collaborators to blackmail, and untold numbers of bounty hunters that combed the land and forests hoping to find partisans or Jews. I keep my deepest secrets to myself. I became conditioned to secrecy, and have been so all these years, even to the present day. It's hard when your life depends on your own voluntary actions. It's easy when secrecy becomes an involuntary habit, and like any deeply ingrained habit, it's almost impossible to change."

On another visit, Paul appeared to be morose and melancholic. I was unprepared for the near-revelation about a crucial aspect of his real-life survival story.

"My days are numbered. My health is failing. During the war, I did some terrible things, but I believe that I've been a good person. So let me share a story with you that I have never shared with anyone. It's about an action that you might appreciate more than others because of your faith."

Then he stopped for a minute, and continued in a rush, "I'm sorry. I'm hesitant. I'm having flashbacks or just bad memories about informers and reprisals. Maybe the story shouldn't be told. Let me defer the grim details. Perhaps another time."

I did not press the point. Several months later Paul was hospitalized with an episode of heart failure that required intensive care and monitoring. He improved slowly. On morning rounds, he was comfortable. I reassured him that he would recover. As I prepared to leave Paul's private room, he asked me to return in the evening because he had "something to tell me." So, I did.

"One early winter day my young son, Leopold, ran into the house as excited as I have ever seen him. He told me that he spotted two adults with a child warming themselves by a small fire in the woods and added that he was not detected.

"Leopold guided me to their location. The threesome had not left. I recognized them even though they were in a huddle to stay warm. They were

Jewish merchants from the village that I traded with over many years. They were trustworthy and honest. Isaak Swartz was unshaven; Leah was holding their heavily bundled infant child. As I approached, both looked downcast and either trembled from fear or from the cold chill of winter. They finally recognized me. This was a dangerous situation. I had no time to linger.

"Stay hidden in the vicinity. Tonight I will return to help you.

"When they nodded in agreement, I wasted no time in leaving with Leopold. That night I could not find them. Finally they emerged from the woods when assured that I was alone. I brought them to my barn, fed them and had them wash. Righteous people of the village had been hiding Isaak, Leah and infant Benjamin a long time. They and other members of their extended Swartz family had been passed from household to household. The villagers knew that Germans were arresting all Jews, were confiscating their property and possessions, relocating men, women and children to ghettos where the strong were forced into slave labor. The others, including the elderly and the children were often murdered.

"When it was rumored that the Germans planned to raid the village in search of political enemies and Jews, Isaak and Leah's extended family split up. Each child was entrusted to a relative. Perhaps some would survive. Isaac and Leah left with their youngest child hoping to join some partisans in the forest. After superficially penetrating beyond the periphery, they became exhausted."

Paul had learned too much and had done enough for the moment. He gave the fugitives some provisions, pointed from whence they came and told them, "Go back to your campsite. I will return in two or three nights and help you."

Once again, Paul stopped and looked about his hospital room with unfocused eyes. He whispered, "What could I do, Doctor? I had to help them even though my plan placed us all in triple jeopardy. Two years after the Germans invaded, Hitler imposed the death penalty for anyone who helped a Jew in even a trivial way. If I were caught helping this Jewish family, it meant a public hanging for them, for me and for my family. There are those who collaborate with the Germans. How am I to know who they are? They might be a so-called trusted friend or a sinister neighbor with ever-watchful eyes. If the Jewish couple were discovered and implicated me, all would be lost."

Paul was committed to help, but needed his wife's approval before moving forward. She agreed to assist the hunted couple and child, knowing that she and her son and in-laws would also be executed if exposed.

Paul explained, "We are religious, God-fearing people. Before our priest was arrested, he told us that this war is God's punishment for our collective sins. We should love our neighbor as ourselves, God is merciful, and peace will soon be restored."

Several nights later, Paul had his rendezvous with the family Swartz.

Isaac asked, "How will you save us?"

"Underground."

Isaac needed clarification, "Do you mean you will guide us to the partisans, to the underground rebels?"

"No, you will be safe underground."

Paul blindfolded the puzzled couple, and then guided them to the emergency shelter that he had held in reserve for his own needs. The shelter was a natural cave carved out of the side of a hill. The main chamber was about ten feet high by forty-five feet deep and ninety feet wide. The roof and walls were supported by wooden and metal beams. The earthen floor was covered with straw. Within, there were stacks of warm clothing, some military-style sleeping bags, cases of wine, smoked packed meats, dried fruits and vegetables—including many stacks of mushrooms. There was an adjacent small chamber that served as a latrine with a lime pit surrounded by a very wide diameter and very deep, thick, steel waste tank filled with lime-covered sand. The cave could be illuminated with smokeless oil lamps. There were stacks and stacks of paraffin oil. At the side of the cave, diagonally opposite the latrine, was a vertical, hand-powered water pump that tapped into an underground stream. The cave was fitted with inconspicuous air vents and an elaborate and marvelous camouflaged crawl-space entrance that could be tightly covered by a huge round boulder supported on wooden tracks that resembled fallen tree trunks. A large jack could raise and lower the tracks by manual cranking from within the interior of the cave or from the exterior entrance. When the tracks were raised, the boulder rolled away from the entrance; when the track was lowered, the boulder rolled forward and closed the entrance. An interior canvas curtain blocked exterior daylight in one direction and lamp light in the other.

When the blindfolds were removed from Isaak and Leah, they were speechless for several minutes. They appeared to be in awe and were overwhelmed as they took in their surroundings; dimly lit by two oil lamps that Paul hung on wall pegs.

Paul spoke: "To remain here, you must agree to three conditions."

Paul then elaborated that the interior crank handle would be taken from the cave, essentially imprisoning the Swartz family. The risk of their leaving and being apprehended was too great. The next condition would require immediate action if the Germans discovered the cave and gained entrance. Isaak and Leah would face sure death after being tortured to name their benefactors. To avoid torture, certain execution and the same fate to their helpers—they must agree to take cyanide immediately upon discovery. Last, they must temporarily give up their infant. The future is too uncertain. Rations and fresh water might become scarce with resupply uncertain. They must agree to have Benjamin placed in the village convent with Mother Superior. She would take Benjamin as she had taken and protected other innocent Jewish children. They were being treated well alongside the many Christian children orphaned in the wake of the terrible war.

"Your son will have a better chance of survival there than here, especially if he has not been circumcised or becomes ill. I will be back tomorrow night. If you agree to my conditions, I will take your child, leave some cyanide tablets and intermittently return with fresh supplies."

The next night, all conditions were accepted. Paul left the tablets and took Benjamin to the convent. With good luck, he would be reunited with his parents at the end of the war.

Paul paused. He appeared to be exhausted as he relived his stressful tale; he drank water from a paper cup and continued his story.

It seemed that God was long on retribution and short on benevolence, for the hidden Jews remained underground for two years. Somehow they maintained their sanity. Food became scarce and their bodies became thin.

As the war wound down, the Germans hurriedly withdrew to defend the Father Land.[2] The next day the brutal Russian "liberators" entered. They were living off the land. They took everything that the Germans left.

"The Russians took our animals and our produce; they took over our homes to billet their soldiers; they took all of our help for their purposes. All captured Germans and any remaining able-bodied Polish men and women were sent to Russia or Siberia for slave labor. We hid out of sight after they took all we had. The resistance fighters avoided the Russians and I would not release our rapidly failing Jewish cave dwellers to them."

Paul was elated when at long last, an American Army liaison platoon came by. The Lieutenant Commander spoke a little German.

Paul became animated when he told me, "Between his German and my English I learned that the Russians had liberated a death camp at Auschwitz. Jews, Poles, women, children, Gypsies, priests and political prisoners had been gassed in great numbers. Basically, almost anyone who was not essential and could not perform heavy labor was executed."

After a pause, Paul continued, "I told the commander about the hidden couple. We went to the cave with a medic and some liter bearers, because I knew that they could not walk far after their long confinement. Isaac had a beard that flowed to his waist. Leah could only support herself for a few paces at a time. The commander ordered that they be gathered up and immediately sent to the Army Medical Field Station."

Paul and his family joined the partisans, then went to a displaced-persons camp and finally to the United States under sponsorship by his church.

After Paul finished his story, he looked directly at me.

"Now I've told you what I have not told anyone else. I'm not really sure how I survived the war. I saw what I hoped I would never see. I learned what I hoped I would never learn. I did some things that I never imagined I could or would do. I believe that it was God's will that I survived and that I was able to help others to survive.

"You are the only one that knows about my Polish-Jewish neighbors. Now that the secret is no longer a secret. I rely on you to keep that confidence.

"Even now, forty years later, as an old man and ill, I no longer worry about myself. I worry about Isaak, Leah, and Benjamin. Did they survive? Were they reunited? I do not know and will never know."

End Note

1. Germany and Russia were secret allies at the beginning of WWII. They became enemies when Germany invaded Russia. That is when Russia and the US became allies against their common enemy—Germany.
2. During the war, the Nazis referred to Germany as the Father Land.

CHAPTER TWELVE
Weddings

Introduction

People commit their loyalty and lives to each other for varied reasons and in many ways. Cultural, religious and individual preferences usually prevail and determine the format. In some societies, marriage is sacred; in others, not so. In some societies or belief systems, the traditional relationship must be between a man and a woman. The union should result in childbirth to perpetuate the blood line or to perpetuate the family name. In other societies or belief systems, marriage can be a nontraditional union.

In the course of a career, physicians observe, or care for, patients who are directly or indirectly impacted by high-grade complex emotional stresses such as hesitancy about moving forward with a commitment, or retreating from one; such as jubilation at the prospect of a long-term relationship, or seeking parental approval before finalizing a plan.

I have witnessed couples who have lived together for years, then marry to honor an ill parent who was hanging on just to see that blissful day.

I have observed a predator woman insist that she marry a wealthy man who was on his death bed—a man that she barely knew.

I have seen an unattached divorcée with her former husband's estranged young son barge into their respective ex-husband and father's hospital room where he was soon to die. The event sent a shock wave into the room. The former husband and present wife had to call security to evict the interlopers, who "only wanted to express well wishes as a measure of their concern and devotion." When the dust settled, the poor guy told me that his former wife had set the stage to challenge his will.

I have witnessed an Intensive Care Unit nurse answer the phone and tell the caller that the patient I admitted the prior night with a heart attack was doing well. And then added, "And by the way, his lovely wife just left after a prolonged visit." The caller replied, "What? I'm his wife!"

There are near endless observations between couples that I have been privileged to witness. Illness brings out the best and worst of human dramas. At the extremes, they can play out as comedy or as tragedy.

This section will detail several stories of patients that reflect relationships within the "Human Condition."

Tradition

I always deemed it an honor to look after a colleague, or a member of his or her family. Doing so defines the platitude, "A Doctor's Doctor." The medical issues are usually complex. If they appear to be straightforward, an unanticipated complication invariably appears.

On an autumn day in 1983, while walking along a hospital corridor, I was approached by Ben Silverstein, a trainee who was starting a rotation in the Coronary Care Unit. I assumed that he wanted advice, a so-called "Corridor Consultation," about managing a problem patient. I was wrong. He asked if I would see his father, Solomon. Ben related his dad's concerns. According to his father, the problem was new-onset chest pain that was reviewed at Johns Hopkins in Baltimore, Maryland. The cardiologist was uncertain of the problem's cause or its gravity. Perhaps I could provide clarity. I agreed.

The next day, Solomon called my office. He was instructed to gather his records and let us know when he would be traveling to see me. I would meet him on a Saturday morning and leisurely review his medical complaint.

That too came to pass. Ben introduced his father then withdrew to finish caring for his patients. Father and son were strikingly similar in appearance. Each was tall and slim, with a high forehead, wavy black hair, full face, large ear lobes and a broad smile with a large space between their two front teeth. We settled into our chairs facing each other. The chairs were positioned less than an arm's-length apart.

"Well, Mr. Silverstein, tell me about your chest pain."

"Please, just call me Sol."

"Okay Sol, tell me about your chest pain."

"I don't have any chest pain. I never had chest pain."

"Sol, perhaps I was misinformed by your son. You didn't send or bring your medical records, so tell me what symptoms you had at home in Baltimore."

"I didn't have any."

"No symptoms, Sol? Then why are you here?"

Sol paused in deep thought. He sneezed. I offered him a tissue.

"It's personal."

"Sol, if it's not medical you don't have to tell me. If there's no medical concern, let's skip the history and the examination and just pass the time. If we don't, Ben will wonder why we spent so little time together. There's a coffee dispenser in the waiting area, let's get a cup and just talk."

I then put my pen and notepad in the top desk drawer.

My cup was dark roast and tasted great. Sol spoke first.

"You know my son?"

"Yes"

"Do you know him well?"

"Fairly well."

"Then let me tell you about him. He is smart, very smart, because he is disciplined and has an ability to focus without distraction. Do you know why he can do that?"

Without waiting for me to answer, "No," Sol went on without a pause.

"It's because he started his formal education in Jewish Day School. A long day spent with secular and religious subjects. That required discipline, concentration and commitment to master each subject. By the time he was ready for college, he was well prepared, very well prepared. So he got letters from elite colleges that said they wanted him and they would give him a full academic scholarship. Do you know why they did that?"

Again, before I could answer, Sol pressed on.

"They wanted an outstanding scholar—it all happened because he went to Jewish Day School."

Sol went on to explain that elite medical schools contacted Ben with the same proposal. They wanted him and offered a full academic scholarship. The reason was the same. They wanted an outstanding student and the reason that Ben was outstanding was simple. He had attended Jewish Day School. Before Sol rested, he invoked exactly the same logic for Ben's current presence at an elite training program in medicine.

So I asked, "Then, why are you here? Why did you fabricate a reason to be here?"

When there wasn't an immediate answer. We both raised our cups and drank. Sol then asked a question without answering mine.

"Do you know Dr. Christine Waterman?"

"Yes, she is a trainee here, just like your son."

"Well, now that I am sure you know her, I'll tell you why I'm here. But, only if you assure me that you are my doctor, you consider me to be your patient, and our relationship guarantees that what I tell you will remain confidential."

"Of course, Sol. You have my word."

When our eyes met, he said, "I trust you."

And then he said, "Parents guide their children. The process is tricky. Too much guidance inhibits self-determination. Too little guidance invites bad outcomes."

Sol paused; he starred into his half-filled cup while organizing his thoughts.

"My Ben has known Christine for some time and my wife and I have met her on previous visits here. They seem to be romantically inclined. My wife and I have never had a religiously mixed marriage in either of our families. Why am I here? At times I feel duty-bound to dissuade my son from pursuing Christine—by the way, what do you think of her?"

"Sol, you might not agree, but I believe that she's intelligent, has a great deal of compassion for her patients, is cheerful and will be a terrific doctor. I like her."

"I like her too. I'm conflicted. That's my problem!"

There was a knock on the door. Ben had arrived to collect his father.

A Matter of Honor

The year was 1969, the time was late evening and the place was the Emergency Department at my inner-city hospital. Bill Chan, a 62-year-old, Chinese, hard-working importer-exporter had been toiling over invoices after hours, when he experienced severe chest pain, nausea and perspiration. He was well enough informed about the symptoms of a heart attack to snuff out his cigarette and take an aspirin before coming to our hospital.

Mr. Chan was the oldest of his three living siblings and when nearly overpowered with chest pain, immediately recalled his younger brother's recent massive heart attack and death. Two remaining brothers and a sister managed the family's prosperous restaurant in the "Chinatown" section of the city. That district had the highest concentration of Asians and Asian businesses.

Bill Chan was relieved when I told him that his attack was minor with only a small amount of heart damage. I assured him that, unlike his brother, survival was expected. It is important to remember that in 1969, heart-attack patients were confined to bed rest and were insulated from exciting news or events. Television and radio news was banned. Death notices were removed from newspapers to allay fears that a friend or relative's name might appear during the critical period of recovery. Hospital confinement for a heart attack ranged between two and four weeks, at the discretion of the attending physician. The minimum was two weeks. Bill Chan was a businessman who understood financial benefit and financial risk. In matters of health he relied on professionals, was compliant for the most part, asked a minimum of questions and was content to be monitored in the Coronary Care Unit.

Some patients are devastated by a prolonged stay in the hospital and others at the prospect of being isolated in a hospital for two weeks.

I remember a man with a probable heart attack who was persuaded to enter the hospital against his instincts. He was the principal of a one-man, barely profitable talent agency. Because of minor concerns, his hospitalization extended beyond two weeks. The agent's artists went to competitors for job opportunities and his business failed.

Another man refused to be admitted because he was a piece worker on an assembly line. He pleaded, "This is my busy season. I earn fifty percent of my income during the next few weeks. My family will be ruined if I don't go to work. I promise I will return to the hospital when the factory slows down."

The medical facts were clear. There was an acute heart attack which carried a 20 percent chance of death. The socio-economic facts were also clear. The man signed out of the Emergency Department, "Against Medical Advice."

I visited Mr. Chan each morning and evening. We discussed the need to rest, to avoid placing undue demands on his healing heart and the need to pursue healthy heart habits such as weight loss, smoking cessation, adequate sleep and exercise.

After five days of discussing medical and other issues with Bill Chan, I learned that he was the family patriarch. His father was long deceased and his mother was cared for by the family. During visiting hours, some family members were consistently the first to enter and the last to leave their patriarch. Apparently there was an impending wedding and the need to modify the protocol if Bill Chan could not attend.

When he asked, I mentioned that, according to the conventions of the day, the risk would be too high, convalescence would be shortened and healing might be incomplete. He countered, "I must attend. The bride is my niece, the daughter of my deceased brother. The groom's family owns the most well-known Chinese restaurant in the city. The wedding would not only be a marriage between two people who are deeply in love, but also an alliance between two families and their business interests."

Before I could reply that his health was more important, Bill Chan closed with a powerful argument.

"As the oldest son and family patriarch, it is my responsibility to represent my deceased brother at the ceremony—it is a matter of honor."

After further discussion, I fully understood that the benefit of maintaining family honor and status in the community was more important to Bill Chan than the risk to his health. However, I did not fully understand his absolute confidence that all would be well when he participated in the ceremony. The wedding day had been selected with great care. The analysis sought an auspicious time that coordinated the best numerological dates of the Chinese calendar with the couple's birth dates, a day that their Zodiac signs were harmonized and a day that the stars would be properly aligned. It would be a great day and Bill Chan believed that his health would be a beneficiary of the day.

On the wedding day, I granted Bill Chan a twelve-hour leave of absence from the hospital for a "family emergency," advised him to proceed at a slow and deliberate pace, and assured him that I would remain in the hospital until he returned.

In the late hours of the night, Bill Chan returned to the medical unit in good spirits. True to his prediction, he felt fine. This honorable man was grateful that he was not forced to sign out of the hospital against medical advice, grateful that I understood his predicament, and grateful that we would maintain our friendly relationship.

In a sense, the wedding celebration was a "movable feast." As a token of his appreciation to our staff, Bill Chan was accompanied by a relative who brought trays of Chinese banquet food on a cart. He was directed to the break room on the cardiac floor where he prepared a feast and invited everyone to partake.

Hospital personnel work in a high-stress environment that is conducive to a high rate of "burnout." So we were appreciative of Bill Chan's gesture. It provided a light moment to counterbalance our constant exposure to the serious consequences of illness.

Damaged Goods

Mary Lou Bell and Anthony Davis were like two ships passing on a foggy night. They were raised and lived in the same community. At times, they both sat in my office waiting room on the same day, but never had sequential appointments. During winter, each couple migrated to the same town in Florida. That had been the annual custom prior to the death of a spouse, and continued to be the case for Anthony, the surviving widower "snow bird." The widow, Mary Lou Bell, had established her permanent residence in Florida, and remained there for the previous five years. She was under the medical care of local Florida-based physicians, whereas, the widower, Anthony Davis, maintained our long relationship. He remained under my care. Mary Lou Bell and Anthony Davis first met when they were introduced by a mutual acquaintance in Florida. She had an attractive youthful appearance with the help of cosmetic surgery and strove to improve her skills as a landscape artist and classical pianist. Mary Lou had an active social life. When asked by a woman friend and confidante to reveal the secret of her popularity with men, she whispered, "It's not my mediocre artistic talents. When I'm with a man, what I do—I do well."

Anthony was a wealthy retired hedge-fund manager who appeared to be physically fit by adhering to a weight-maintenance diet, attending a class of supervised comfort-level exercises at a gymnasium three times each week and playing recreational golf.

Both Mary Lou and Anthony had had the good fortune to be in a long-term happy marriage. Each had been the primary support of their spouse during illness. Each became exhausted as they watched their spouse being ravaged by a progressive and prolonged disease—" 'Til death do us part."

After their spouses's death, both Mary Lou and Anthony were drawn to each other by the unpredictable mysterious forces that guide human behavior. Perhaps Anthony had a need for companionship to dilute his loneliness. Mary Lou was not wealthy, had no children and perhaps desired a long-term secure relationship. Within a brief period of time, their friendship intensified. They were often seen together in public and were seldom apart in private. The relationship morphed into a romance. Anthony's New England-rooted children anxiously sensed that their father's romance might lead to matrimony. Anthony and Mary Lou hadn't known each other one full winter season. Anthony's children wondered if their father's heart was controlling his head, for he would never make an important hedge-fund decision without a quarterly report. Winter hadn't run its full course; less than one season was less than one financial quarterly statement.

Each party involved in a romance might overstate an attribute in a bit of deception with hopes of appearing highly desirable in the eyes of the object of their affection. As Mary Lou and Anthony accelerated their commitment to each other, I later learned that Anthony spent lavishly and engaged in some "false advertising." I will never know if Mary Lou exaggerated her situation.

In early spring, the couple secretly became engaged and decided to announce their intent to marry when they came back to New England. Their return was delayed when Anthony became short of breath and had evidence of fluid retention. During an overnight visit to the local Florida hospital Emergency Department, the problem resolved after excess fluid was removed with diuretics. There was no time for a followup visit because the couple was scheduled to fly to New England the next day. Anthony's discharge instruction was to call his doctor for an appointment when he arrived at his destination, or go to an emergency room if his symptoms returned. There was no mention of eliminating salt from Anthony's weight-maintenance diet.

On the evening flight to Boston, Anthony impressed Mary Lou with spacious first-class accommodations. The dinner menu was unexciting. There was nothing special on the standard or vegetarian fare. However, the Kosher choices, available to all, were more to their liking. The chicken soup appetizer and boeuf bourguignon entrée were appealing. The meal was outstanding, but highly salted. As a consequence, symptoms of fluid retention returned. After deplaning, Anthony barely made it out of the airport, went directly to the hospital as directed, and was admitted under my care. His weak heart had required my guidance through several prior hospitalizations.

Mary Lou was anxious. How could Anthony, a perfectly healthy man by his account and appearance, rapidly deteriorate before her eyes?

During a family meeting that included Mary Lou and Anthony's children, I explained that Anthony had a decade-long history of progressive heart weakness. He had been on heart medication for years. He would survive the current crisis, would be stabilized on more potent medication but would not possess his previous level of energy and vitality.

The information was readily accepted by the adult children. Because of past crises, they were aware of their father's heart condition and its guarded long-term outlook. Mary Lou, on the other hand, was incredulous and shaken. She sat absolutely still, but could not prevent her hands from trembling. Then her eyes narrowed and she frowned. She stood, and in a soft, almost inaudible voice, murmured, "We had plans— We had plans."

Then in anger: "He lied to me. He lied about his health and perhaps his wealth. He wanted me to be his nurse. I did that once and won't do it again. Tell him 'goodbye' for me. I'm out of here."

Her last words trailed behind,

"All along, the bum was damaged goods."

CHAPTER THIRTEEN
The Good Death

Introduction

When I was a pre-teenager, I went to religious services with my family on the Jewish High Holidays. At that time, I took the written word in scripture literally rather than metaphorically.

There is a passage that every person's fate is determined for the coming year.

"Who shall live and who shall die."

The possible circumstances and types of horrible deaths, and only horrible deaths, were enumerated. Death by fire, drowning, the sword, starvation, thirst, earthquake, plague and strangulation were among the options. Scary stuff. I concluded that it was best not to stray from the path of righteousness. Perhaps that was the intent of the passage.

At a later time, I wondered why there was no mention of placid deaths, sudden painless deaths or heroic deaths; when in fact there are a myriad of possibilities.

During my medical career, I witnessed varied forms of death. Some were agonizing, most were controlled, some were sudden, the majority were painless, and all were sad — for a life had been lost forever.

The stories that follow are examples of how some patients respond when they have time to direct their possible or predictable death.

Contemplating an Honorable Death

How we die can be important. The majority of earthly creatures have no choice. Death can result from natural causes, accidental causes and wounds sustained in warfare. A minority of sick people have options. Such was the case with Boris Brass. He was a retired medieval scholar whose most threatening past health problem was coronary disease. He had experienced several minor heart attacks, and currently had intermittent chest pains. His heart condition was a reminder of an uncertain future. But when Boris thought of dying he was consoled by the fact that his legacy was ensured by being an international expert in medieval history and an author of several highly acclaimed books.

Boris was now 83 years old with thinning hair, a wrinkled face, failing eyesight and twisted arthritic fingers. He was a long-term widower, his children lived abroad and he currently enjoyed the solitude of puttering about his home—a mansion that was situated in the center of fifteen acres of wooded grounds and walking trails.

Boris had long been troubled by the prospect of dying from a heart attack. He was living in the twentieth century, but his mindset was often in the fifteenth century. To his amazement, he had exceeded the average age of an Englishman living in the fifteenth century by fifty years. Boris believed that he should have died long ago from any one of his heart attacks.

Those added years not only promoted poor vision, but also enlargement of his prostate gland, which is a common problem of elderly men that prevents the urinary bladder from completely emptying. Time is not a friend. The progressive increasing amounts of residual urine that remain in the bladder promote urinary tract bacterial infections, that further promote inflammation and ultimately causes further obstruction of outflow. Relief occurs when the bladder is drained with a catheter tube. Antibiotics are always required.

Boris had several dangerous infections from bacteria that entered his blood stream (sepsis) and caused high fever, very low blood pressure and near cardiovascular collapse. During each attack of sepsis, there was the possibility of permanent organ failure and death.

I remember a decisive day when Boris was in the Intensive Care Unit recovering from a near miss with septic death. He was a typical, critically ill, intensive-care patient attached to a web of electrical wires that led to and from a variety of machines and catheter tubes of all types attached to his aged body.

I entered the room, sat at the bedside, looked directly at him and greeted Boris.

"Good morning, I hope that you are feeling better today."

"I recognize the voice of my long-term cardiologist. Let me put on my spectacles to be sure. Yes, it's you. Let's get serious."

"Serious, about what?"

Boris then explained that he would likely die from another attack of sepsis caused by his enlarged prostate gland. The problem could be cured by a relatively uncomplicated operative procedure to reduce the blockage of urine that flows through the prostate. The operation would lower the possibility of future urinary tract infections, but the operative risk could be a severe, if not fatal, heart attack.

There had been several previous discussions between Boris and his urologist surgeon about the benefits and risks of undertaking the procedure. Few surgeons would accept an invitation to have a patient die from a heart attack during an elective operation to prevent recurring urinary bladder infections.

So Boris was in double jeopardy. He faced the prospect of dying from urinary sepsis, or undertaking a surgical procedure that could trigger a fatal heart attack. Boris believed that the time had come to decide when and how he might perish, rather than leave the matter to chance.

"My choice is easy," he explained. "Some deaths are noble and others not so. The death certificate of the Voodoo Queen of New Orleans reads that she died from 'Diarrhea.' Imagine. That's expected of a peasant, but not a queen."

The way that Boris saw it, dying from a heart attack was far more noble than dying from a urinary infection. So, Boris chose surgery and the urologist acquiesced to his wish for an operation.

A Socially Acceptable Death

I was introduced to many of my patients while they were caught up in a life or death struggle. For them, I strove to be a reliable and constant presence; a life buoy in a turbulent sea. When the storm passed we were tightly bonded as patient and doctor. For, I too was part of that immense contest, as I made every effort to guide my patient to a safe harbor.

I met Murray Mueller when he had a heart attack caused by the excruciating pain he experienced while passing a gallstone. When he stabilized, further heart studies revealed generalized coronary disease. Medications and a heart-centered lifestyle program were immediately initiated to retard further progression of coronary narrowing.

Murray had detrimental health habits. He was a two-pack-a-day cigarette smoker, enjoyed fried fast food, was sedentary and was an angry man. His psychiatrist could not undo his anger and depression with "happy pills."

My patient was a Certified Public Accountant and tax specialist who could not hold a position worthy of his training and experience for more than a year. Fortunately, Murray was hired as a bookkeeper by a relative who was in the home-heating business. Twice divorced and estranged from both former wives and his only child, Murray was 64 years old and was counting the days to retiring at 65. Work and the simple requirements of living were confounding burdens, so much so that Murray was incapable of boiling an egg or toasting a piece of bread.

Appearing older than his age, this misfit's head was in constant motion which caused his long white hair to flop about. His facial pallor was striking; eyes of blue darted about; and his stout hands constantly trembled. Mentally ill with chronic depression, and unable to generate a thought that might cause a ray of brightness to penetrate the gray gloom of his mind, there were no good days or expectations of having a better tomorrow.

Unable to find solace, Murray's anger intensified at having a gall bladder with stones that would cause pain during their escape, a heart with blocked arteries and the prohibition of his two comforting rituals—smoking tobacco and eating at fast-food franchises.

Murray and I got to know each other well during the six months following his heart attack. He reluctantly ate healthier meals, exercised and lost weight. His blood pressure and cholesterol improved on this regimen, but his depression worsened because each intervention towards improving physical well-being was a reminder of his mortality. Murray became preoccupied with morbid thoughts, so much so that he started to plan for death. Legal documents were prepared. Worldly possessions were given to charitable causes. Pre-paid funeral arrangements were made. The only unfinished business was to actually die.

"Doctor, I never want to suffer the pain of another gallstone—never."

"We previously spoke about risky gall bladder removal, but I believed that your heart was too shaky to tolerate the stress. Now that you're responding to our medical program, if your next cardiac exercise test improves, perhaps you can have your gallbladder and stones removed."[1]

"I don't want to wait. Can't you just prescribe an overdose of pills that'll kill me?"

"If you want to die from an overdose, why don't you empty all the bottles of your medication and overdose yourself?" (My question was unethical.)

"I can't take an overdose because my religion would mark me a sinner. Suicide is forbidden. I've already asked for forgiveness for my sins and expressed remorse for my past bad behavior. I've received prayers for the sick. I'm fully prepared to depart. Why can't you help me with some pills?"

"Well Murray, my religion, and all those that I know of, forbid murder."[2]

"Oh. I was mistaken; I thought you were an atheist."

"Even if I were, medical ethics and natural law forbid murder."

I informed his psychiatrist of our discussion. Another cardiac stress test was performed. When I noted that the test had improved, Murray insisted on having his stone-filled gallbladder removed even though there remained a chance of an intercurrent catastrophic cardiac event.

Murray told the surgeon that he would undertake any and all risks to avoid having another excruciatingly painful stone passage, pancreatitis, or gall bladder perforation. The surgeon informed Murray that the operation carried a moderate to moderately high risk of a complication or death.

The surgery was scheduled. A cardiac anesthetist was put in place, and medications were administered to reduce cardiac strain. Murray was grateful for our cooperation. He assured the surgeon that whatever the outcome, it was his fully informed choice to go ahead with the operation. He would accept full responsibility for a bad outcome and absolve the entire healthcare team if such were to occur.

The operation was successful and without complications. The heart was well behaved throughout the procedure. A rock-solid performance.

During my first post-operative visit, Murray was still partially under the influence of general anesthesia, and mistook the gowned nurses for heavenly angels. During my second visit, he was fully conscious. His unexpected greeting was, "You bastard, you said I would die during the operation and I didn't."[3]

End Notes

1. During this timeframe, non-invasive gallstone-removal technology had not yet been introduced.
2. When a physician refused to commit euthanasia at a suffering patient's request he was told by the patient, "Don't worry, I won't tell anyone." Jennifer Kay. Clifford Irving at 87; published a fake Howard Hughes book; Boston Globe. December 23rd, 2017; B8
3. Some patients hear what they want to hear rather than what is said. My primary intention was for a successful operation. Murray's primary intention was to be a fatality in the course of surgery, and thereby have a socially acceptable death rather than death by suicide.

A Good Doctor and His Good Death

For decades there has been a national trend for deaths to occur in hospitals or healthcare institutions rather than in a home setting. The majority of hospital deaths occur in an Intensive Care Unit with its technology-dense environment of physiological monitors, intravenous machines, arterial oxygen recorders and respiratory ventilators. Many patients are on life supports that have prevented their death. Some will recover, many will not. Some have already died but present the illusion that they are still among the living because their chests rise and fall in unison with ventilator-mediated lung inflation and deflation. Hearts that have ceased to beat are artificially stimulated with an electronic pacemaker. Chemistry and fluid balance is maintained by an artificial kidney for those poor devils whose natural kidneys have failed. The wrecked unsalvageable bodies of the should-be-dead are nourished with intravenous or tube-fed nutrients. When life supports are compassionately removed, the result is certifiable death.

Whenever possible, the medical establishment respects the wishes of patients regarding their tolerance for life-normalizing or life-saving discomfort.

For any number of reasons, some individuals choose to end their painful or painless lives, rather than to be a burden to others. When I was on the consulting staff of a residential nursing home, an occasional ancient patient would stop eating, refuse medication and not drink. Without an apparent dollop of daily pleasure, they often said, "I have lived too long." They uniformly claimed to have nothing good in their future except an interminable delay of a desired natural death. Ultimately, some had a revelation that they had the power to induce their own painless and peaceful death in a manner that would solve their problem of merely existing. So with few ways to exercise control, they simply refused to take medication and nourishment. I had no direct or indirect involvement with these residents. I was merely an observer.

At a much later time, I had the privilege of witnessing and interacting in the "good death" of a wise and compassionate doctor who had been blessed with a long and productive life. As a young man, he had thoughts of committing to a spiritual life, as had some of his forbearers. Then he considered a career in the arts, perhaps music. Finally he chose to be a physician, an academic and an investigator. He rose to a high rank, then emeritus when he reached age-based retirement. The good doctor's body needed intermittent repairs, yet his mind remained youthful and his memory exquisitely sharp.

After the death of his wife, the good doctor lived alone and even when a centenarian, remained fully independent and active. He regularly attended the symphony, the theater and medical meetings, and he frequently memorialized colleagues and friends. In time, he personified Oliver Wendell Holmes' metaphor of being the last remaining leaf on a tree.

At home, the good doctor was busy keeping abreast of the medical literature, performing computer searches in areas of personal interest, listening to music from his extensive collection of recordings and enjoying works of art that covered the walls of his home.

Life had been full. The journey had been long. What would occur in the yet to be determined short term? Likely loss of independence, loss of control and loss of self-determination. With predictable troubled times ahead, the good doctor decided to let his life slip away. After informing his family of his decision, he stopped taking all medication and nourishment. While filling his home with music, the wise doctor exchanged private thoughts with visitors, former patients, neighbors and friends from his many communities. I was welcomed at the bedside as one of his caring physicians and as a friend from the medical community.

When death took him from our midst, the good doctor died an artful death as it might have been in ancient times prior to the practice of scientific medicine. The elements were being at home surrounded by family and community, having an awareness of imminent death and being comfortable as life ebbed.

I believe that the wise doctor orchestrated his own "good death."[1]

End Note

1. The good doctor was a student of medical history. He was likely aware of the ancient concept of *ars moriendi* (the art of dying) and his need to modify some of its requirements. https://en.wikipedia.org/wiki/Ars-moriendi

CHAPTER FOURTEEN
Regrets

Introduction

This book is a collection of remembrances. Each patient has a unique story. I have tried to weave the threads of several individual patient experiences into a composite patch of fabric that can be viewed through the lens of empathy and compassion. The sum of many patches represents the quilt-themed larger story of this book when clinical care had not surrendered its patient-centered mission to a business model that demands rapid processing of valuable commodities represented by patients who have profitable financial value. Current medical-business practices are causing career dissatisfaction among healthcare professionals because their patient load, chart-documenting requirements and oversight do not permit enough time to know their patients. Many physicians and nurses are experiencing high levels of workplace stress and "burnout."

In the beginning, organized medical care was for the sole benefit of patients. Currently, there are too many scandalous media reports about patients having unnecessary tests, procedures or treatments for the sole benefit of entities within the medical establishment.

Fortunately, the leaders who guide many institutions of healing are extending a helping hand towards the personal needs of their workers and patients.

Even in the best of times, there were outcomes that were unsatisfactory, unanticipated or disastrous. None were caused by physician-related error.

What follows is a trio of stories with regrettable outcomes that continue to trouble me.

Unintended Consequences

I erroneously believed that Janet Stover would be a routine consultation. She was a 78-year-old lady with a heart murmur. Her diagnostic cardiac studies revealed that she had mild narrowing of the aortic and mitral valves. The beginning of the aorta (main artery) was moderately calcified. Her medical history revealed kidney stones, loss of height from 68 to 64 inches and an elevated blood-calcium level. I wondered if an overactive parathyroid gland (hyperparathyroidism) had been overlooked. I ordered a parathyroid hormone level. When it returned substantially elevated, I instituted a referral to an endocrinologist. The more interesting aspect of Janet was her social history. It was so unusual that some would swear she was born under a lucky star.

From day one to old age, Janet had good luck. She was born and raised in Virginia, of caring parents. Each of their prosperous families was deeply imbedded into Southern aristocracy. Her early education was at exclusive all-girl parochial schools. When she was eighteen, she was presented at a coming-out ball with her cohort of "sisters" to formalize their being marriage eligible. Yet Janet was committed to other goals before she would consider marriage. The most important was to learn about attitudes that differed from those of her Southern culture; to experience different viewpoints—such as the liberal views in some parts of New England. After high school, she intended to go to Boston for her continuing education.

Janet was an attractive brunette with hazel eyes and a smile that exposed pearly white teeth. Young men fantasized that she had "inviting" red lips. She had a healthy complexion, an engaging personality and a slim five-foot-eight body that disguised its strength. Janet was a powerful woman. She could hike trails for miles, could climb moderate mountain heights and was an equestrian who could fully control a nine-hundred-pound horse.

As Janet was possessed of a creative mind, a retentive memory and a gentle, persuasive manner, her parents yielded to her plan to travel to Boston to attend college if she could satisfy three conditions: she must go to an all-girls school, she must only date Christian caucasian boys, and she must return to Virginia upon graduation.

The first condition was the highest hurdle to overcome. Would an elite greater-Boston all-girls college consider an applicant from a small Southern parochial school? Janet applied to Jackson, Radcliffe, Wellesley and Regis College. She was accepted to all, and matriculated to Radcliffe, class of 1925. She was content to study only as hard as needed to achieve a passing grade. Her purpose was to receive a liberal education that would challenge her rigid Southern societal structure. An active social life developed with men from varied co-educational and all-male colleges in the vicinity. True to her agreement with her father, all of her escorts were fine gentlemen of the Christian faith.

In her third year, she married Marcus, a recent graduate of Boston College, with excellent prospects in his family's food-marketing business. By choosing to withdraw from Radcliffe, Janet officially became an attendee, rather than a graduate of Radcliffe. By the letter of the agreement, rather than its spirit, her non-graduate status permitted Janet to remain in New England.

Massachusetts was among the first states to legalize prohibition. Abstinence was not an agreed-upon requirement of attending college in Boston. The city was replete with speakeasy bars and nightclubs. A popular spot was the Pickwick Club in Chinatown. On July 4, 1925, Janet and her husband were at the club to celebrate Independence Day. The festivities extended beyond midnight. At 2:00 A.M., 200 patrons (a number that exceeded the legal capacity of the club) were stomping on the dance floor to the music of the Charleston, when the rear wall of the building collapsed. Janet and her husband heard what they believed was a delayed volley of fireworks, but the floor suddenly tilted and sharply sloped towards the black night where the back wall had been. She slid out of the building with other revelers just as the upper floors collapsed like a stack of pancakes and crushed many of the unfortunates who remained.

Janet's fall was broken when she landed on a pile of moaning patrons. She bounced off, righted herself and walked away as structural debris and screaming revelers rained down. Marcus also escaped unharmed. Janet's lucky star was shining bright that night.

By another stroke of good fortune, Janet had a happy marriage, raised three children and had two robust grandchildren when we first became acquainted.

When the diagnosis of hyperparathyroidism was confirmed, we had two management options. They were medical therapy with the prospect of medication-related side effects, or surgical removal of the parathyroid glands that are situated above each half of the thyroid gland. I assured all parties that Janet's heart should be able to tolerate curative parathyroid surgery. An endocrinologist would manage the immediate reduction in calcium generation and adjust the dosage of artificial parathyroid hormone.

During the operation, an expert surgeon was only able to identify and remove three of the customary four parathyroid glands. The continuous elevation in calcium levels indicated that the fourth gland was active and hidden. Special scans located its anomalous location within the left lobe of the thyroid gland. "Fortunately," a new catheter technique could locate and block the blood supply to the wayward gland, which should then atrophy and cease to function in the aftermath.

In the course of the blood-supply ablation procedure, the catheter brushed against a calcified atherosclerotic plaque on the inner wall of the calcified aorta. A piece of plaque broke off and was transported up the left carotid artery to the dominant left hemisphere of Janet's brain. The damage resulted in a major assault on her being. She was no longer independent, no longer with vitality, no longer able to speak or think clearly and no longer with self-determination. Her luck had run out. Her lucky star had imploded and its light extinguished. Many patients in her situation would prefer to die. Each of her doctors, including me, would choose to turn the clock back and follow a different path.

After absence of neurological improvement, the final blow came one week later. The cardiovascular stress from the surgery and the stroke caused a fatal heart attack. A standard surgical procedure resulted in a horrible outcome about which I have regret upon regret. Janet's life journey was ironic. She escaped a building collapse where 42 people perished and 100 were injured, but died from complications of a very low-risk operation. No one was prepared for her death. She never said "goodbye" or conveyed a last wish to her family. She only demonstrated great faith in her doctors.

Sacrificed for the Greater Good

Mort Greenfield was in the late autumn of his years. His mind was intact, but little else was normal. He had a heart murmur from a narrowed aortic valve. A recent picture of the valve indicated that the narrowing wasn't critical. Adult onset diabetes had nearly wrecked his kidneys, and had so damaged the circulation and nerves in his legs, that his feet were constantly numb. Mort's eyes went dark years ago. In spite of many limitations, he appeared to be a contented, non-complaining man. Just as two plus two equals four, a voracious appetite plus a sedentary lifestyle equals a rotund body. Mort's wife, Nancy, was a major ingredient in the formula for his happiness. She was a decade younger, was in good health, was a strong advocate for her man and was forever caring.

Mort had been a successful senior officer in the Manhattan branch of an international brokerage firm. Years after he retired, the couple moved to Boston to be closer to Sarah, their widowed daughter, and her children. That's when and where I first met Mort, as I had cared for Sarah's husband after he collapsed from a heart attack while in a pedestrian crossing. Mort was "stable" when he and Nancy left Boston to winter at their luxurious home in Palm Springs, California. Five months later, Mort developed progressive fluid retention that appeared in his legs, then his abdomen, then his lungs. The crux of the problem was a combination of kidney and heart failure. The cause of the latter was a surprise. It was critical aortic stenosis, a problem that prevents enough blood to pass through the valve to adequately supply the body's needs for nutrition and oxygen. Mort was told by his California doctors that he was not a candidate for corrective surgery, only a candidate for more-intensive medical therapy that had little prospect for significant improvement.

At the time, I was away from my home base on an exchange assignment at the cardiology department of a neighboring greater-Boston hospital to learn about some leading-edge investigations of new technology intended to benefit valvular heart disease. One new-technology early-phase study was a clinical trial of a catheter capable of stretching open a critically narrowed aortic valve with a balloon, thereby eliminating the need for conventional heart surgery. The new procedure was termed aortic balloon valvuloplasty.

Being wise enough to realize that his days were numbered, Mort was fully prepared for the inevitable. He had lived an exemplary life. Mort was a virtuous person who always respected his fellow man as they traveled through their life journey. He was charitable and was faithful to his religious doctrine and its rituals.

Sarah contacted me in a panic. Her father had improved, but his California doctors offered little hope of survival in the short term. She asked, "Do you have any ideas?"

I told her about the aortic balloon valvuloplasty. When she expressed an interest, I told her that I would speak to the prime investigator and learn if Mort qualified for the study. The answer was, "Yes, pending an exam and further studies when the patient is transferred to our hospital."

With that news, Mort was evacuated on a private medical flight to Boston with high hopes of being put on a path toward a longer life. He told me in what would become a prescient statement, "I know the implications of the fluid that caused my body to swell, that caused my shortness of breath, and caused my heart to pound fast. Doctor, I've had a good life. Thanks for the opportunity to live longer. If things don't work out, I'm prepared for the worst."

Several teams involved in the clinical trial reviewed Mort's status. The heart surgeons declined to operate because of his general high risk and continued heart failure. The aortic balloon valvuloplasty team agreed to perform the procedure because Mort was a fairly good, but not ideal, fit for their protocol. He was high risk for any procedure, but too high a risk for surgery. Of the ten patients who had already undergone the balloon procedure, eight were improved, one was unchanged and one had died during the valvuloplasty.

While Mort's kidney and heart failure were being stabilized for his procedure, there were two patients cued up ahead of him. The first died and the second nearly died after her valve was torn open by the balloon.

The experimental procedure was now in jeopardy of being terminated. So a decision was made to only perform the procedure on moderate-risk rather than high-risk patients. Mort was no longer a valvuloplasty candidate. The administrators of the experimental program had to deny care to some patients in order to benefit the majority. Mort was out of contention. The remaining options were medical therapy or surgery.

Mort was a financial analyst. He and the heart surgeons were schooled in "risk analysis." The surgeons had their program to protect. In an atmosphere of public reporting, too many bad outcomes could destroy the reputation of their program and their hospital. The heart surgeons were asked to review Mort's case again.

The chief surgeon was gentle with Mort: "You're too frail at the moment. If you improve, we'll reconsider your case."

The natural history of critical aortic stenosis with congestive heart failure is the protracted decline of an exhausted heart.

Mort graciously accepted our inability to help him. After thanking me for my efforts, he was discharged to the comfort of his home with an uncomplicated program of oxygen, medicine to eliminate fluid and home-health aides. He died in familiar surroundings.

Although his death might be termed "a good death," I know that he was sacrificed with a Do Not Treat Decree in order to save the clinical trial. I also know that his life might have been extended had the natural progression of critical, valve narrowing been slower. When he was transported from California to Boston, aortic balloon valvuloplasty was an experimental "newborn" clinical procedure. Critical stenosis was detected too late for surgery and too early for balloon valvuloplasty. Not long after Mort's death, the procedure was finally approved. Every high-risk patient with critical aortic stenosis became a candidate for the procedure. No patient was too ill. It was even performed as an emergency for those in cardiovascular collapse who were at the edge of the grave.

I encouraged Mort to come to Boston and still regret that he wasn't at the head of the procedure queue upon arrival. We both had high hopes of a "medical miracle."

Duke

During the Vietnam conflict there was a call for doctors to serve their country. I had a choice of assignments and elected to sign on for a two-year commitment as a Cardiovascular Research Associate at New York's Staten Island Public Health Service Hospital. Career public health officers were permitted to be housed on federal land at, or near, the hospital. I did not have that privilege and had to explore the real-estate rental market. Staten Island had been a tranquil borough separated from the New York mainland by New York Harbor. Access to and from the island was by ferry boat. I arrived 19 months after the Verrazano Bridge connected the island to Brooklyn. Land speculation and a building boom followed. Time was short, demand was high and rental housing was in short supply. I settled on a street-level duplex that was within a ten-minute drive to the hospital. My wife would have made a better selection, but she was busy preparing for the move and attending to our young child. The secretarial staff at the hospital later told me that I inadvertently chose to live among "a pocket of undesirables."

In time, the secretaries were proven to be correct. There were now three routes of public access to and from the island: an old bridge connection to New Jersey, a new bridge connection to Brooklyn, and the traditional ferry-boat connection to lower Manhattan. The long-term residents constantly spoke of the good-old-days before, as they said, "undesirables" began flooding into Staten Island.

The local newspaper was replete with reports of crime. Even we made the news when our apartment break-in and robbery was reported among a dozen others that occurred on the same day. It seemed, from the daily crime reports, that all trucks hijacked within a fifty-mile radius of my new "home" ended up abandoned nearby. The neighbors were colorful. When they learned where I worked, they offered me "hot," hijacked goods in exchange for free health care at the hospital or low-cost groceries and merchandise at the Post Exchange. When I declined, in the back of my mind, there was always a lingering concern about an imminent reprisal.

200   Stafford I. Cohen, M.D.

The research position at the hospital was exciting. I had a great group of co-workers and the science was to understand the electrical system of the heart (electrophysiology). We sought answers to what controls its normal and abnormal beating, the influence of the inner heart on the forces on the outer-body-surface electrocardiogram (ECG), the influence of cardiac drugs on the electrical properties of the heart and how to apply electrical therapies to control abnormal heart rate and rhythm. Experiments were performed on human volunteers and laboratory animals. We worked long hours and had most weekends off, although we usually spent part of each weekend analyzing experimental data.

When my wife and I relaxed at a movie, or went out socially, we had a teenage girl from the neighborhood come to our home to look after our youngster. Terry was a smart girl with a tangle of curly black hair, brown eyes and a big Brooklyn accent. She had abundant experience looking after her multiple younger siblings. A typical teenager, on occasion Terry appeared in heels rather than sneakers, had mascara about her eyes and applied ruby-red lipstick. Terry had a dog named Duke. He was a very large, docile German Shepherd. On some days she brought Duke along when she arrived at our home. Terry's father, Giovanni, or Gio for short, believed that his Terry and our home would be safer with Duke on the premises. Duke arrived with his tail wagging, sniffed or nuzzled my legs and sat after a pat. He had a brown and black coat with unusually striking white markings on each paw and a large white diamond shaped spot on his forehead.

While walking about the neighborhood for exercise, I occasionally went by Terry's house. The backyard was fenced in with a prominent sign that read "No Trespassing: Beware of the Guard Dog." One day I met Gio while passing his house and asked, "Do you have a guard dog in addition to Duke?"

"Nah, when no one's home, Duke guards de back of de house and two large sheds in de yard where I store my merchandise. By the way do yuh need any new tires, a T.V., or liquor?"

When Duke failed to accompany Terry to our home during several of her working visits, I questioned if he was all right.

"Oh, my dad found a new family for him in de country. Duke almost attacked a neighbor's kid who wandered onto our property. Someone left de fence gate open. My dad heard a commotion and run out just in time to call Duke off before he pounced on de kid. The kid's father, Rocco, said he'd poison Duke if he wasn't removed. Rocco's one of my dad's managers, so Dad agreed. I really miss Duke."

With only 16 weeks remaining to complete my research at the Public Health Service Laboratory, I came across an article published by a cardiologist that defined the ECG pattern of an arrhythmia that originated in the left atrium—the left small upper chamber of the human heart. I wanted to confirm that observation by stimulating the comparable chamber of the dog heart. I hoped to nuance the published finding by stimulating the small chamber at its high and low borders and its lateral edges. This acute experiment would require several large animals. A personal request to Jason, our supervisor at the research-animal compound, was all that was needed. I had the willies each time I entered his office because it had a large bulletin board with notes pleading for the return of pets that had been kidnapped or lost. A photo of each pet was attached as well as their name, their habits and an offer of a reward if returned. Jason said that none of the missing had ever found their way into his domain. He assured me that if there were no large dogs under his care, he would contact each New York City borough stray-animal pound or animal-care center where strays or unwanted pets were euthanized if not claimed or adopted within 14 days. So whenever Jason and his staff made a transfer, for one of our acute experiments, they essentially granted a temporary reprieve, rather than a pardon, to those animals already on death row.

While in medical school, my resistance against experimenting on animals softened when I read testimony given in 1948 by heart surgeon Dwight Harken at a public hearing before a Massachusetts legislative committee regarding a proposed anti-vivisection bill. Harken spoke of his experience with four separate groups, each with thirteen similar heart operations and their results. All thirteen died in the first group, seven died in the second, two died in the third group and all survived in the fourth. The fourth group was composed of wounded soldiers evacuated from the European Theatre shortly after D-Day. The subjects in each in the first three groups were laboratory animals.[1,2]

Our early experiments with left atrial arrhythmias went well. The last experiment was scheduled shortly before my discharge from the Public Health Service. Immediately after arriving at my office on the morning of the last experiment, I was beckoned by the program director to review a manuscript before its final submission to a medical journal. Ben, my collaborating partner on the left-atrium-arrhythmia research project, agreed to start without me. Together, we had extensive experience with the protocol.

After a prolonged discussion with the director about last-minute edits of the article to be submitted, I went to the animal laboratory, opened the door and looked about. The oscilloscope before me had six, real-time, high-quality ECG channels streaming across its face.

"Ben, how's it going?"

"Without a hitch."

I glanced at the side view of the deeply anesthetized subject secured to the animal cradle. The open chest had been closed after placement of the four pacing wires on the heart's left small chamber. The chest fur had been completely shaved to secure the ECG recording skin electrodes. They appeared to be properly positioned. The animal had been intubated to control respirations when the chest was opened and during the administration of deep anesthesia. The canine's head was turned away from me. The extremities were secured to the cradle to prevent undue motion. Hum. The two paws in view were white. I circled around to the back of the table that held the cradle. The paws on the opposite side were also white and—and there was a white diamond on the forehead of this oversized German Shepherd.

Damn! This was Duke! How could this be? If I had been there at the start, I would have called it off. My mental agony quickly became physical.

"Ben, I'm not feeling well. Can you carry on without me?"

"Sure thing. You're pale. Are you sure you're all right?"

"I'll be O.K."

On moving day, Gio appeared to wish us well and to thank us for having confidence in his Terry by trusting her with our most cherished possession—our young son. He handed us a brown bag that held a bottle of "his best wine." As he left, not realizing that he was telegraphing Terry's surprise, he mentioned that she would be right along with a batch of her freshly baked cookies. After some hugs, Terry gave us a gift-wrapped box of homemade chocolate-chip cookies. She had become more adult during our two-year friendship. She said that she would miss us, but not nearly as much as she missed Duke.

"My dad says Duke has a lot a space to run around on de farm. He's so happy; it's as if he's in dog heaven."

Feeling my eyes become moist, I turned away.

"Terry, I'm sure he is."[3]

End Notes

1. Harken DE, Harken AH. Commentaries. Anti-Vivisection. Have we waited too long? Arch Surg 1989; 124: 1386-87. In this commentary, Harken refers to his 1948 testimony.
2. Stafford I Cohen. Paul Zoll MD: The Pioneer Whose Discoveries Prevent Sudden Death. Salem, New Hampshire; Free People Publishing 2014: 16-18. Harken's successful heart operative experience with wounded soldiers during WWII is documented and further referenced.
3. I never wished to, or had to, perform another experiment on an animal.

EPILOGUE

Clinical medicine is a Science and an Art. In the remote past, Art shone because there was little evidence-based science.

"The Art of medicine" is practiced when a competent physician takes a complete history and "lays on hands" while performing a comprehensive examination. An empathetic and compassionate physician understands the patient's concerns and feelings, comforts the patient and does something to help.

In recent years there has been an exponential advance in the Science. Now, Science has no mercy—it has suffocated the Art. At all levels, technology needs most of the available oxygen to maintain its trajectory. There has been major progress in basic science, applied science, diagnostics and therapeutics—as well as abundant accessible health information for doctors and patients. In the area of delivery of clinical care, there has been major change with mixed reviews regarding the extent of progress.

In the current climate, doctors must spend many hours documenting the precise elements of each patient encounter—so many hours that they have little, if any, time to apply the Art of medicine in word or action. Doctors now spend about 60 percent of their workday as digital-entry clerks and with non-patient-oriented administrative tasks.[1] The Art is a necessary skill that bonds doctors with their patients in at least a quasi-traditional meaningful relationship. The Art has historically defined doctoring as a unique, noble, and very special undertaking.

Many factors have adversely impacted the traditional delivery of care and the patient-doctor relationship. I will mention some of the factors.

The Electronic Medical Record: A Help and a Hindrance.

The US government allocated 37 billion dollars in incentives between 2011 and 2017 for Internet healthcare.[2] That is approximately $44,000 per Medicare-participating practitioner to incentivize the transition of a patient's paper medical record to an electronic medical record (EMR).[3,4] The EMR is stored in a registry available to all doctors involved in the care of each patient. For efficiency of time and scale, the EMR is generated during a patient's approximate eight-to-fifteen-minute followup office visit. As a result, most of a practitioner's time is spent updating the EMR rather than directly interacting with their patient. Changes in clinical status, medications, social status and other parameters are essential for ongoing care—and must be documented.

Some electronic programs are complicated, prevent nuanced data entries and are incompatible with systems used in other hospitals or offices within or outside of the home network. It is said by many doctors that the EMR is "death by a thousand clicks." Experts acknowledge that entries into the EMR currently take more time than expected. But according to Robert Pearl, a past CEO of the Permanente arm of Kaiser Permanente, the content-time trade-off favors the content. It should be noted that the Permanente arm of Kaiser Permanente spent four billion dollars to install the Epic brand EMR within their large system.[5]

An article in *The Harvard Business Review* comments, after investigating hefty technology, that it is common for healthcare institutions that invest in high-performance technology to have "little to show" for their efforts.[6] Many users of EMR programs believe that they are unfriendly. Some doctors are so frustrated, they are leaving the profession. In a 2013 survey, 12 percent of doctors who had been in practice between ten and twenty years were planning to leave medicine for other non-medical careers.[7] Some doctors are so frustrated and burned out, they are leaving the profession rather than being forced to enter data into an unfriendly EMR program that distracts from giving patients their undivided attention, which was the reason for going into medicine in the first place—to be "with" a patient during their pain and distress.[8] Between 2011-2014, there was accelerated burnout and dissatisfaction among physicians.[9] In Letters to the Editor of the *Mayo Clinic Proceedings* about this phenomenon, physicians attribute the cause to the EMR, micromanagement technology and corporate control of medical practice.[10]

During a patient-doctor visit, there should be a time share between the Science and the Art of medicine—between the doctor's use of technology and the doctor's unencumbered empathetic interaction with their patient.

New discoveries in science and advances in technology must be applauded. They are essential to reverse ill health and to sustain good health. Technology is expensive. Many observers believe that technology is overused by some doctors and institutions to generate income or to establish a defense against a claim of negligence given the realities of our litigious society.[11] In a recent survey of 4,000 practicing physicians, more than half had been a defendant in a malpractice case.[12,13] There are many causes of physician stress such as the weighty responsibility of ensuring the best outcome for a patient, avoiding the sins of omission or commission in the care of a patient and avoiding emotional or physical fatigue. It is estimated that approximately half the doctors and as many allied health workers have experienced some degree of stress-related, generic burnout,[14] a condition that can lead to an error. Even if a distraction-caused error leads to no harm, the very fact that an error occurred can lead to depression or worse. There are 400 suicides a year among US physicians—that is a rate six times greater than other professions.[15]

In the April 2019 issue of *Fortune Magazine*, there was a damning review of the Electronic Medical Record. Patient injuries and deaths were attributed to malfunctioning systems. Dissatisfaction with doctor-patient relationships has been exponentially increasing during the several years that I have been writing this book. Dividing an all-too-brief visit between the EMR and the patient is an impossible task. The number of bad reviews of the EMR far outnumber the laudatory.

Enlightened leaders, managers and administrators at the top tiers of organized non-profit and for-profit medicine must find a way to shield doctors from the ever-expanding onslaught of bureaucratic regulations, to permit them a little more time to be with their patients. If that is not possible, leadership should allow more direct-patient time by speeding data entry on the EMR that provides the best evidence-based approach to disease.[16] Change will not occur from the bottom up. Change must occur from the top down.

The Art of Medicine

The Art of Medicine is all about making the patient aware that their doctor is with them and will stay with them. The Art of medical care is difficult to teach and difficult for students or trainees to learn if they are not innately endowed with a compassionate nature or if during their youthful formative years they did not have empathy and compassion impressed upon them by role models.

Hopefully a student or trainee endowed with these helpful qualities will not let the hectic pace of learning and training diminish or annihilate those beneficial attributes—attributes that define what many patients desire in their physician and attributes that set the superior physician apart from the majority of their mediocre colleagues.

The Science of Medicine

If mediocre trainees become mediocre physicians and teachers, each generation runs the risk of a progressive lower standard of medical expertise and care-based performance.[17,18] Yet, technocrats hope that the shortfall can be partially mitigated by the abundant use of advanced technology that might suggest an accurate diagnosis and recommend the latest treatment guidelines.

I know several master teachers who question the effectiveness of trying to transfer their expertise to the next generation of physicians who will not be given enough time to take a complete history or to perform a comprehensive examination. Given that reality, there will be an erosion of quality of care. One simple solution could be for program directors to set aside protected teaching time and to extend the duration of some, if not all, patient visitations.

It's not too late. History can set an example that a lesson learned is a lesson not forgotten. In the early 1800s, approximately two centuries ago, medicine was long on Art and short on Science. The trend toward Science started in the mid-1800s. Oliver Wendell Holmes, Sr., spent his first two years of medical school in Boston; his mentor was Dr. James Jackson, Sr.

Holmes' last two years were spent in Paris. Its medical schools and hospitals were state run. The full-time professors were selected on the basis of merit. There was an abundance of cadavers—the "passive teachers" of anatomy, and the lectures and clinics were free to foreign students. Furthermore, some physicians of the French School had refined the patient examination to learn the signs of underlying illness. Perhaps the most important advance of the time was the invention of the stethoscope by René Laënnec.

Although diagnosis was improving, medicine was still more an Art than a Science. It would take another 150 years for medicine to become a true science, while the Art still had a preeminent place.[19]

In Paris, Holmes found such a superior level of medical knowledge and understanding of illness that he wrote that the worst doctor on the staff of École de Médicine was better than the best doctor in America: "...where stupidity is tolerated, where mediocrity is applauded and where excellence is deified."[20]

Holmes latched on to Pierre-Charles-Alexandre Louis as a mentor. Louis had developed a scientific numerical system of classifying a patient's symptoms, signs and organ pathology, if and when there was a death and autopsy. All the information was placed in a registry, much the same as registered medical information is mined today. Louis' scientific method was valued in contrast to the biased opinions of others. Louis' intense scientific approach to disease was believed at times "...to be greater than his interest in curing the patient."[21]

When Holmes and other American disciples of Louis returned home, they became zealots for the scientific method. Yet in his old age, Holmes questioned his unconditional devotion to Louis. In retrospect he had undervalued his original mentor James Jackson, Sr.'s artful, compassionate and comforting approach to each patient.[22]

In the spirit of Holmes' late revelation, I believe that the Art of medicine should be preserved in what remains of the 21st Century. At the bedside or in the office, a physician must learn about the patient as well as their illness.

The Commercialization of Medicine

What are the projections for the delivery of medical care in the remainder of the 21st Century? With the help of advanced technology, we race to eliminate disease and prolong life at low cost per patient unit. The process should not be labor intensive. Efficiency should shave many hours from many a physician's excessive schedule. Sounds good! But the time-saving technocrat visionaries do not address how medical leaders and administrators will re-allocate those vacant hours. Those hours must be designated a purpose. Past and present technologies are promoted as time-savers. Yet, most doctors continue to work excessive hours. Many doctors are in a constant state of sleep deprivation and fatigue. In all likelihood those vacant hours will be filled with more patients added to each doctor's existing, overflowing panel. Medicine has become a big business. One in eight Americans are employed in the healthcare industry, or, in other terms, 16 million job descriptions support 50 million people.[23] In business, "time is money." Administrators cannot leave money on the table. Norton M. Hadler, M.D., an academic investigator and clinician who finds fault with the many ways that the business model of our current medical health-delivery system has devalued the patient-doctor relationship, once wrote, "Today, health is a commodity. Disease is a product line. Patients become units of care. Physicians become production workers."[24] Perhaps as a matter of institutional self-interest, more administrators will extend office visits and offer varied opportunities to reduce stress in the work force.

Might Future Scientific Medical Developments Further Harm the Patient-Doctor Relationship?

Visionaries that specialize in the distant future of our health believe that all aspects of disease will ultimately be revealed from specific cellular DNA, biochemical markers, pathophysiological correlations and clinical presentations. Massive amounts of data will be gathered, stored, mined and categorized, with hopes for new discoveries,[25] rather than failure to do so.[26] Medical information doubles at a minimum rate of every five years and will be available to knowledgeable machines as small as a smart phone that can interact with a physician, with a patient or with other machines.[27] With the help of intelligent machines—termed virtual assistants—a doctor might be able to manage an enormous case load. Prototype virtual assistants are currently being marketed.[28] It is speculated that machines will be able to directly interact with a patient and diagnose and prescribe in the same manner as their supervising doctor. In time, the intelligent machine might resemble the doctor—might almost be a copy of the doctor—but, unlike the doctor, the machine could work unlimited consecutive hours without making an error attributed to fatigue.[29]

If these predictions come to pass, nurse practitioners, physician assistants, certified health coaches, scribes and some doctors could become endangered. Their roles replaced by intelligent machines that will be far more advanced than Siri and Alexa. Such predictions were made in 2013[30] and again in 2017.[31] Artificial intelligence today may not appear to be a powerful transformer, but advocates advise that paradigm shifts take time. Early in 2018, the Food and Drug Administration approved artificial intelligence software that could be used to identify wrist fracture, diabetic retina eye disease and the identification and treatment of various strokes, without a specialist necessarily confirming the software's diagnosis. Before long, artificial intelligence will overtake expectations.[32,33]

With data in hand, a doctor-patient interaction can be brief. In theory, an intelligent machine can take the history, sort out the subtleties and generate a short list of possible diagnoses. Another machine can perform the diagnostics such as analyze blood, sweat, urine, saliva and exhaled air. The physician will have a hand-held ultrasound imaging machine that can look into any part of the body. If there is pathology, the doctor can prescribe an intervention. If surgery is required, it might be performed by a robot with a "steadier hand" than a surgeon.

Sounds good, doesn't it? But who will program the intelligent machines? Who will categorize and separate the massive core of medical data into bins? Who will synthesize the data? Who will be the masters? Will programmer bias be eliminated?

Raymond Kurzweil is a proven visionary in the field of artificial intelligence. While currently working with Google, he predicts that in the next several decades there will be unprecedented gains in the war against diseases such as heart and lung conditions, cancer and microbial infection. They will be understood and will be well managed. Longevity will be extended to as much as 120 years. Kurzweil even envisions that an avatar of his deceased father could be created from a currently stored sample of DNA and his father's written thoughts committed to journals, diaries and other documents.[34]

Well, how will these predictions impact the doctor-patient relationship? Will the unique humanistic aspect of doctoring to others continue to be of value or be replaced with another paradigm of caring to be delivered by machines that have intelligence, but no true feelings of empathy or compassion? If so, will there be a way to preserve a doctor-patient relationship built on trust? I hope that the administrators charged with framing the delivery of care by the medical establishment will value the patient-doctor relationship, and that the social engineers and economists will permit the time for a compassionate doctor to vet the concerns of a needy patient. I hope that the framers of policy will include the opinions of physicians in their deliberations. Even the physician CEO of America's largest health-delivery network scheduled additional office time to bond with needy patients.[35]

During a newly announced healthcare initiative that will structure the care of more than one million workers, surgeon Atul Gawande, its leader, included improving patient-doctor relationships among his goals.[36]

A recent article in a premier medical journal raised the possibility that advanced medical technology could significantly decrease the need for patients to directly see their doctors. Telemedicine visits, diagnoses across computer screens, and wired or wireless communication all could serve busy patients and busy doctors. This business model is admittedly driven by entrepreneurial providers, who want to succeed in gathering marketshare. With that kind of technology, a patient's complaint can be taken care of by telemedicine without the need to drive to a medical office that has the technology on site; and doctors are left more time to do "what only we can do."37 Well I ask: Why are so many doctors and patients dissatisfied with the current system and its uncoupling of patient-doctor interactions? What is it that "only clinical doctors" can do? Aren't they trained to care for patients; to interact directly with patients; to determine a course of action after speaking with, and examining a patient? Sorting out an in-person medical complaint shouldn't be a second, third or last resort!

Unintended Problems with an Aging Population

What about the dying? If lifespan is extended in the future, there should be a comparable extension of youthfulness, self-determination and quality of life. If not, suffering will be prolonged and nothing will be gained.

What about those who currently, or in the near future, are about to have a relatively slow death—those who will not benefit from the prediction of remarkable scientific discoveries in the future? What about those patients who do not believe in a providential God or do not believe in an afterlife in Heaven or Hell? Some believers and non-believers with terminal illness want the option of physician assistance in preparing to die. They want the option of selecting the time and place to depart by their own hand with physician-prescribed medication. To choose to die from the natural progression of their fatal disease or to self-terminate their physical or emotional pain and suffering along with their life.

Some foreign countries and jurisdictions within the US have laws and regulations that permit a physician to prescribe a lethal combination of medication to terminally-ill patients who qualify after meeting defined standards. The prescribing physician must avoid being present during the patient's final act, if indeed the patient fills the prescription and decides to take a lethal dose. There are currently about seven US state jurisdictions with enacted legislation that permit physician-assisted death with medication. The laws are known by several labels: Death with Dignity, Physician Assisted Suicide, Medication Assisted Suicide, Medical Aid in Dying and Compassionate Choice. I will use the label Compassionate Choice to emphasize that physicians and terminally-ill patients, in conscience, can choose to participate or not participate in legalized programs. For the patient, there are three timeframes for choice. The first is to choose to participate, or not to participate in the program. The second moment is to fill, or not fill the prescription. The third moment is for the dying patient to take the lethal combination of medicine, or to return it to the medicine cabinet. Furthermore, a physician also has a choice to participate, or not participate in the program. Physicians that subscribe to the program are exempt from prosecution as long as they are absent during their patient's final earthly act. A physician's presence, in any way, at that time would qualify as euthanasia, or, to use another term—murder.

Some relatives of terminally-ill patients that died while being attended to by palliative care or hospice programs told me in as many words, "Society treats our suffering pets better than our fellow humans who are suffering with a fatal illness; who have short-term prospects of living, but must endure severe and prolonged agony."

Society permits euthanasia for animals dying from natural or accidental causes. Horses do not recover from a broken leg. I witnessed such a tragedy during a training session at Saratoga Race Course in upstate New York. The injured horse was given a lethal injection by the racetrack veterinarian and quickly succumbed.

In another context, US federal jurisdiction and some state jurisdictions permit taking a death-row convict's life. The US Constitution's Eighth Amendment states that the death penalty should be administered in a manner to terminate life without purposefully harsh or unusual pain or suffering. So the garrote, firing squad, beheading and hanging have been eliminated. The electric chair had its day. Lethal injection is the present method. Physicians, who honor the ancient Hippocratic oath to do no harm, will not directly participate in any aspect of an execution as a matter of conscience, and the American Medical Association has a similar prohibition. While the US federal judiciary, and the judiciary and citizens of some states condone the death penalty, the opponents of Compassionate Choice might be asked, "If our government and a portion of our society permit its convicts to die quickly and painlessly, why not offer the same end-game to all citizens with a fatal illness?" A fatal illness has served its host with a death notice. One symptom is often intolerable pain. To the sufferer, each day is much longer that 24 hours.

A physician has two missions, to cure illness and to comfort the suffering. There is a strong trend for more jurisdictions in the US to legalize Compassionate Choice. Citizens are aware that the relief of terminal pain is a high-wire balancing act. Too little medication does not relieve pain and too much medication consciously or unconsciously can result in an overdose death—and a charge of euthanasia. I foresee a groundswell of jurisdictions opting to assist the dying that choose to end their suffering with the help of their physician. The issue will require many conversations between patient and doctor. It will be of an intensity that cannot be duplicated by a machine. A machine that lacks true feelings cannot relieve suffering better than an empathetic compassionate doctor. I do not foresee those qualities in a futuristic machine.

Conclusion

A recent article by C.A. Colaianni documents her grit, forbearance and resilience while enduring physical hardship and illness during a surgical training program.[38] She referred to Robert Scott, the Antarctic explorer, who also endured hardship in pursuit of his goal to be the first person to reach the South Pole. In response to the article, Dr. Ammu Susheela and I wrote that Roald Amundsen, an experienced Norwegian explorer, beat Scott in a race to the South Pole. Scott's death and those of his comrades while returning to base camp was the result of poor planning. Amundsen took a shorter route, relied solely on dogs to pull light sleds, travelled on skis when possible and had superior frigid-weather body and foot wear.

Currently, too many deliverers and recipients of health care are dissatisfied with the system. There is a disconnection between a caregiver's goal and their ability to know their patients. For well documented reasons, too many doctors and nurses suffer from "burn-out," leave the profession or commit suicide. Administrators must find a way to create a less arduous trek —as did Roald Amundsen.

The doctor-patient relationship is a unique interaction between humans. So let us hope that this relationship can be fortified, will be valued and will endure. Let us strive to have truly compassionate physicians and health professionals enter and remain among the ranks of those who, with unswerving loyalty, administer and deliver care to the medically needy.

End Notes

1. Mass M, Fisher KA. Why your doctor's computer is so clunky. The Wall Street Journal; March 21, 2018: A15
2. Sasni NR, Huckman RS, Chigurupati A, Cutler DM. The IT transformation health care needs. Harvard Business Review; November-December 2017:130
3. Robert Pearl, MD. *Mistreated.* Why we think we're getting good health care—and why we're usually wrong 2017; Public Affairs: 197
4. Wikipedia. Electronic Medical Record
5. Nortin M. Hadler, MD. *By the Bedside of the Patient* 2016; Chapel Hill. The University of North Carolina Press:133
6. Sasni NR, Huckman RS, Chigurupati A, Cutler DM. The IT transformation health care needs. Harvard Business Review; November-December 2017:130
7. Dyrbye LN, Varkey P, Boone SL, Satele BA, Sloan JA, Shanefelt TD. Physician discomfort and burnout at different career stages. Mayo Clinic Proc 2013; 88(12):1358-1367
8. Priyanka Dayal McCluskey. Complex Partners computer system brings a prescription for frustration. The Boston Globe; May 17, 2016:A1
9. Shanafelt TD, Hasan O, Dyrbe LN, Sinsky C, Satel D, Sloan J, West CP. Changes with satisfaction with life-work balance in physicians and the general working population between 2011 and 2014. Mayo Clin Proc 2015; 90(12):1600-1613
10. Letters to the Editor. Mayo Clin Proc 2016; 91(4):536-537
11. Shanfelt TD, Dyrbye LN, Sinsky C, Hasan O, Satel D, Sloan J, West CP. Clerical burden and characteristics of electronic environment with physician burnout and professional satisfaction. Mayo Clin Proc 2016; 91(7):836-848

12. Henry Marsh. *Admissions*. Life as a brain surgeon 2017. New York, NY; Thomas Dunn Books. St Martin Press:160
13. Medscape Malpractice Report 2015: Why most doctors get sued. www.medscape.com/features/slideshow/public/malpractice-report-2015 cites Krupta C. Medical liability: by late career 61% of doctors have been sued. American Medical News; August 16, 2010. http://www.amednews.com/article/20100816/profession/308169946/2/#cx (This web site is not functioning. The entire article might be obtained from The Center for Justice and Democracy.)
14. Shanfelt TD, Dyrbye LN, Sinsky C, Hasan O, Satel D, Sloan J, West CP. Clerical burden and characteristics of electronic environment with physician burnout and professional satisfaction. Mayo Clin Proc 2016; 91(7):836-848
15. Robert Pearl, MD. *Mistreated*. Why we think we're getting good health care—and why we're usually wrong 2017; Public Affairs: 197
16. Mandl KD, Kohane IS. Escaping the EHR trap—The future of health IT. N Engl J Med 2012; 366:2240-2242
17. Herbert L. Fred. *On Medicine Today* 2014. Friendswood Texas; Total Recall Publications, Inc:15-29
18. Nortin M. Hadler, MD. *By the Bedside of the Patient* 2016; Chapel Hill. The University of North Carolina Press:45
19. Lewis Thomas. *The Youngest Science* 1983. New York, NY; Bantam Books:11
20. Morse JT. Oliver Wendell Holmes volume 1. New York, London; Chelsea House, 1980:108-09. A reproduction of the original book. Boston and New York. Houghton, Mifflin and Company. The University Press, Cambridge. 1896.
21. David McCullough. *The Greater Journey* 2011. New York, NY; Simon & Shuster Paperbacks:126

22. Holmes OW. *Scholastic and Bedside Teaching.* Medical Essays 1842-1882. Houghton, Mifflin and Company, Boston and New York. Cambridge: The Riverside Press; 1839: 305-306.
23. Nortin M. Hadler, MD. *By the Bedside of the Patient* 2016; Chapel Hill. The University of North Carolina Press:112
24. Nortin M. Hadler, MD. *By the Bedside of the Patient* 2016; Chapel Hill. The University of North Carolina Press:145
25. Robert Pearl. The David and Goliath of health care: Apple's Siri Vs IBM's Watson. Forbes/Pharma & Healthcare; October 3, 2013
26. Casey Ross. When it comes to health decisions, Watson hasn't been much help. The Boston Globe. June 18, 2018: B9-10
27. Robert Pearl. The David and Goliath of health Care: Apple's Siri Vs IBM's Watson. Forbes/Pharma & Healthcare; October 3, 2013
28. Priyanka Dayal McCluskey. Virtual assistants lend ear to doctors. The Boston Globe; January 10, 2018: A1, A9
29. Norman Winarsky. What AI-enhanced healthcare could look like in 5 years. https://venturebeat.com/2017/07/23//what-ai-enhanced-healthcare-could-look-like-in-5-years/catagory/ai
30. Robert Pearl. The David and Goliath of health care: Apple's Siri Vs IBM's Watson. Forbes/Pharma & Healthcare; October 3, 2013
31. Norman Winarsky. What AI-enhanced healthcare could look like in 5 years. https://venturebeat.com/2017/07/23//what-ai-enhanced-healthcare-could-look-like-in-5-years/catagory/ai
32. Steve Lohr. A.I. today may underwhelm, but before long it may overtake expectations. The New York Times; December 1, 2017:B3
33. Casey Ross. Artificial Intelligence is evolving fast, but can the FDA keep it up? The Boston Globe; June 11, 2018: A1, B9
34. Herman W. Jenkins. Will Google's Ray Kurzweil live forever? The Wall Street Journal; April 13-14, 2013: A13

35. Robert Pearl M.D. *Mistreated* Why we think we're getting good health care—and why we're usually wrong 2017; Public Affairs: 280
36. Felice J. Freyer, Janelle Nanos. New Health Care Company to be based in Boston. The Boston Globe; June 21, 2015; A1, B14
37. Duffy S, Lee TH. In-Person health care as option B. N Engl J Med 2018; 378:104-106
38. Colaianni CA. Terra Nova. N Engl J Med 2018; 379:19

Stafford I. Cohen graduated from Brown University and pursued his medical training at Boston University School of Medicine. He has been a licensed physician for 51 years, working for most of his career as a cardiologist at a medical center in Boston. He has authored and co-authored many articles and research studies, published in peer-reviewed medical and scientific journals as well as newspapers and book chapters. His previous book is: *Paul Zoll, MD: The Pioneer Whose Discoveries Prevent Sudden Death.*

Dr. Cohen can be reached at:
staffordcohen@gmail.com

www.ingramcontent.com/pod-product-compliance
Lightning Source LLC
Chambersburg PA
CBHW021357210526
45463CB00001B/132